SpringerBriefs in Child Development

For further volumes:
http://www.springer.com/series/10210

Daniel F. Shreeve

Reactive Attachment Disorder

A Case-Based Approach

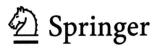 Springer

Daniel F. Shreeve
The Carilion Clinic
Rehab Building
2017 South Jefferson Street
Roanoke, VA 24014, USA
danlshreeve@yahoo.fr

ISSN 2192-838X   e-ISSN 2192-8398
ISBN 978-1-4614-1646-3   e-ISBN 978-1-4614-1647-0
DOI 10.1007/978-1-4614-1647-0
Springer New York Dordrecht Heidelberg London

Library of Congress Control Number: 2011939063

Printed on acid-free paper

Springer is part of Springer Science+Business Media (www.springer.com)

Acknowledgments

I would like to thank my colleagues at Kennebec Behavioral Health Clinic in Waterville Maine, also at the Carilion Clinic in Roanoke, Virginia for their advice, suggestions, and encouragement during this project. I owe a particular debt to Gary Curtis, Child Psychologist, at Carilion Clinic for his critical reading of my manuscript and for his many helpful recommendations. For her excellent and steadfast support of the literature review, I am grateful to Jane Burnette, Hospital Librarian at Carilion Roanoke Hospital. I would also like to thank my wife Marikje Shreeve, Advanced Practice Nurse in Psychiatry, for her professional review of the many drafts, as well as for her patience and inspiration throughout the process of writing and revising.

Contents

Chapter 1
Introduction

Format of the Exercise

This exercise introduces the clinician to reactive attachment disorder (RAD), a childhood disorder involving a general failure of social relationship caused by early, grossly pathogenic care. In order to begin a study of such fundamental impediment to attachment in earliest life, we must as students of child psychiatry define what we mean by "attachment" and also must consider how we will prove a relationship to emotional neglect. A brief introduction to the process of normal, early childhood attachment is essential, before turning to the definition of abnormal attachment and to the topics of differential diagnosis and comorbidity.

Our representative case of "Jorge" is presented as unfolding over time and structured to illustrate challenges of diagnosis to show examples of overlapping syndromes and to promote reflection on what questions may arise during treatment. Within the case presentation are additional, brief segments – identified as "case points" – which bring in topics related to treatment of RAD so as to add a degree of dimensional realism to the illustration of clinical method. An initial set of test questions follows the case presentation, to enliven the exercise.

A review of the etiology of RAD is necessarily broad and interdisciplinary. Adhering to the biopsychosocial model, the section on etiology will cover current theories divided into "biological basis," "psychological factors," and "social origins." Sections which follow the case presentation serve to illustrate, within limits of space available, the directions of advancing research. One example of the unknown, for instance, is how the experience of deprivation at critical stages leads to RAD for some children, whereas others overcome even severe disadvantage. A related, and equally unanswered question, is whether our definition of secure attachment as "normal" actually matches with the history of our species, a history characterized by rare periods of peace and frequent episodes of violence or extreme adversity. Recent work on the adaptive advantage of a range of attachment types is presented, as a prelude to further questions about "what we are treating."

D.F. Shreeve, *Reactive Attachment Disorder: A Case-Based Approach,*
SpringerBriefs in Child Development, DOI 10.1007/978-1-4614-1647-0_1,
© Springer Science+Business Media, LLC 2012

We return to the topic of the principal role of the psychiatry clinician within an interdisciplinary system of care, in the final sections on treatment of RAD. Many methods of therapy have been applied to this difficult disorder, and the summary is necessarily brief. The section on psychotherapy follows conventional psychiatry categorization into evidence-based treatments, those with professional consensus, and those without evidence which may do harm. A second test on general principals follows, and there is an explanation of answers at the end of the text.

By completing this exercise the interested learner should be able to:

1. Define attachment behavior in terms of early mother–infant interaction and explain the evolutionary significance of attachment in the species, as well as relate disorders of attachment to psychopathology
2. Define reactive attachment disorder (RAD) including subtypes, with explanation of the origin and what is generally known about longitudinal course
3. Define the subtypes of attachment as characterized by Ainsworth and others, and compare these to RAD
4. Explain major theories of the etiology of RAD and relate them to the explanations for human diversity in the types of attachment
5. Recognize common comorbidity of RAD and envision how to participate as a psychiatrist on an interdisciplinary treatment team with a real case

What Is Attachment?

Attachment is so familiar to most of us – so basic to social life – that we may rarely perceive it to be an option. When one reflects on one's own relationships, past or present, attachment cannot be defined as something fixed or immutable. Even for close bonds, the sense of attachment recedes one day, and advances the next. Strictly speaking, attachment is also not equivalent to attachment behavior [1]. The presence of danger, for example, provokes attachment behavior, but when the environment is constant the attached ones – child or adult – may draw apart physically or emotionally for a time, perhaps to verify independence, or to gauge the degree of intimacy. Thus attachment itself is a predisposition rather than a behavior. It derives as an accretion of shared moments, such that new events are interpreted in the context of past co-experience. Even when apart, a mental conversation may continue, or the story of a separate adventure is prepared for telling.

We may thus adopt a working definition of attachment as a selective interest in an individual with whom we share new experience with implicit reference to the past together, and whom we will miss if unable to communicate about our responses to something new. Perhaps attachment is best understood in emotional terms when it is interrupted, as we experience distress or longing for the missing loved one. This makes reactive attachment disorder (RAD) all the more difficult to accept in a child, since we would expect a normal dependency on adult figures, related to the need for relatively greater protection in early life. We therefore turn next to the definition of original authors of attachment theory, whose writings comprise the basis for understanding RAD and its treatment.

The Place of Attachment in Nature

An exploration of emerging new theories for RAD may best follow our approach to an example that illustrates the approach to a real case. To assess psychopathology, however, we need a model of normal attachment, and we will review a developmental model of normalcy, which has guided clinicians and families, both at the stage of assessment and in treatment.

Often referred to as "the father of attachment theory," John Bowlby [2] considered both humans and other primates and the conditions of survival. While a psychoanalyst by training, Bowlby embraced the important advances of ethology of his time and sought to apply this natural science, founded in evolutionary theory, to the science of human attachment. Attachment behavior, from an ethological perspective, is any action of infant or mother that promotes proximity, the essential condition for human safety in the wild. As summarized by Main [3], the infant separated from his attachment figure(s) will usually lose food, water, warmth, shelter, and protection from predators.

Bowlby [2] defined stages of attachment for the mother–infant dyad, beginning with the first 3-month period of indiscriminate orientation response to the proximate sources of comfort. In the next several months, the infant recognizes and develops a preference for one or more familiar caregivers. An important influence on the next stage – from late in the first year through the third year – is the growing ability to ambulate. This gives the child some control over proximity, and conversely there is an advancing capacity to explore the surround, using the mother as a "secure home base." Mothers, as part of the "attachment system" favored by evolution, closely monitor the toddler's advances in independence, as well as state of need, especially need for rescue in times of distress. For this stage, theory of natural selection predicts that fitness of the child increases with appropriate balance of safety and exploration, whereas biological fitness of the parent increases in proportion to sensitivity to the infant's immediate state of need.

The following stage, as recounted by Bowlby, involves the child's growing awareness of the mother's mood and direction of interest, such that a "directed partnership" emerges. A mutual sensitivity to signals and familiarity with the pattern of reciprocal responses yields a certain familiarity in this earliest example of human relationship. A biologically coded capacity for attachment is shaped by particular shared experiences of parent and child.

Building upon Bowlby's theory of attachment, Ainsworth and her colleagues developed a typology for attachment in childhood [4]. Ainsworth and Bell [1] theorize that the purpose of prolonged infancy in our species – and the adaptive value – relates to the human capacity to explore, and the importance of an extended supervision of the exploratory phase "a prolonged infancy would miss its adaptive mark if there were not also provisions in the genetic code which lead the infant go be interested in the novel features of his environment – to venture forth, to explore, and to learn." Of equal value to proximity-seeking is thus the exploratory urge, involving also the parent's flexible appraisal of progressive independence; "at first infant and mother are in almost continuous close contact, soon they are in collusion to make more elastic bonds that unite them."

Ainsworth is perhaps best known for her design of a laboratory test that defines types of attachment, beginning with the primary divide between secure and insecure types of attachment. The Ainsworth test for child attachment type – the Strange Situation – is a structured sequence of separations from and reunions with the caregiver (with and without the examiner present). Imbedded in this sequence are the critical reunion episodes, which reveal the nature of the mother–child attachment. A securely attached toddler will freely explore the environment when their mother is present, shows moderate distress at separation, and then will show immediate, obvious joy on reunion. Insecure toddlers in contrast delay their greeting of the returning parent, turn and move away, or even show tantrums when the mother returns to the room. A further subtype of disorganized attachment reveals itself at reunion in a mixture of approach and withdrawal responses, contradictory emotions of high intensity include expressions of neediness, aversion, and angry resentment [5].

In the middle-class American population studied by Ainsworth and her colleagues, secure attachment had the highest frequency, around 60% of the sample. As regards the pathological significance of insecure attachment, Ainsworth did not rush to conclusions. For example, she did not claim (contrary to some viewpoints) that insecure attachment is a direct function of parenting errors. Nor does Ainsworth propose a direct relationship between difficult temperament and disorganized attachment. Perhaps because of this careful science, the Ainsworth typology and the Strange Situation test itself remain useful in ongoing empiric research on attachment behavior in young children, and have been applied to the study of RAD. It is important to note however that RAD is not a subtype of attachment nor part of the Ainsworth typology; it is more accurately defined by relative absence of selective proximity seeking. For clinical purposes, a chief complaint or primary problem in RAD is the impairment in selective, progressive, and exclusive relationship.

The Process of Attachment in Early Childhood

Two events during infancy life, related to our subject of attachment, have critical effects through the lifespan: emergence of a sense of self and the growth of a capacity to regulate emotions. Mahler's seminal work on separation-individuation in early childhood [6] proposes a series of stages in the construction of the self: from earliest infancy an "autistic" self-absorption transitions to a stage of symbiotic merger, or oneness with the mother. The stage of "hatching," at around 5–9 months is the earliest point of separation-individuation, following which, during the "practicing" stage (9–16 months) the child practices independent actions always relying for potential rescue, or emotional reassurance from the parent figure while advancing the zone of independent enterprise. Practice in independent exploration supports individuation, whereas availability of the parent figure allows for an internalization of a model for resolution of distress. Reliability of the parent figure in the face of emotional storms also reinforces a belief in the "other" as a constant, dependable, and separate individual. Mahler's concept of "the psychological birth of the human infant" thus entails a dawning awareness both for self and for "other," each as a differentiated individual and hence ready to interact.

Countless episodes of separation and reunion lead up to a stage of "rapprochement," the point at which – roughly 16 months and older – the infant must reconcile the urge for independence with a growing awareness of the risks of separation. Adventuring away from the parent figure seems to lose its quality of pure adventure and celebration, and may even involve the infant in an appearance of sadness, which may concern the parent [7]. Yet this more conscious comprehension of individuation comprises the essential model for "relationship"; the dyadic relation now involves self, other, and their variable transactions. With the recognition of separateness comes fear of abandonment and a sense of loss of the earlier state of union with the loved one. Success in the infant's struggle for separation-individuation requires the internalization of a model of self and a model of others as authentically separate. As defined by Mahler, object constancy – achieved in the third year – is a "capacity to recognize and tolerate loving and hostile feelings toward the same object; the capacity to keep feelings centered on a specific object; and the capacity to value an object for attributes other than its function of satisfying needs." The conceptualization of self and other is the platform for a real attachment model for subsequent relationship beyond the dyad.

Certain qualities in the caregiver may be crucial to successful individuation. As defined by Winnicott [8] the "good enough parent" is one who is empathic toward the infant and available to assist the child's moment-to-moment, purposeful actions. An example of such "facilitated gesture" might, for example, start with the parent attending to their child's effort to reach for a toy which is too high up, and then their own action to bring the object just into reach. Opposite to this is Winnicott's "substituted gesture," an action by the parent that interferes with the purpose of the child, as driven by the parent's own, and separate aims. An example could be the parent who persistently urges a child to sustain an activity or theme when they are clearly fatigued, or when they have shifted to a new interest. Winnicott depicts the "good enough parent" as providing the "holding environment," within which the child can advance to a definition of self. But, with potential relevance to RAD, in the absence of empathic parenting the child may strive to conform to the adults "substituted gesture." The child's accommodation to adult substitution of motive can give rise to a false self [8]. A possible application to RAD is an appearance of "pseudomaturity," defined as a show of self-sufficiency which seems to eliminate the need for parental help or intervention [9].

Equally pivotal to our understanding of our first attachment is the concept of attunement described by Stern [10], according to which the parent identifies with the child's immediate state of emotions, such that the reciprocal responses of parent and child transpire with emotions implicitly shared in the moment. Attunement is an identification with the emotional state of the other, which recognizes and validates a co-experience of the moment and, through this sharing, reinforces the centrality of the dyadic relationship. Attunement also vitalizes and energizes the dyad, producing a kind of dynamic force which energizes the engagement of parent and child [11]. Tronick [12] proposes that in secure attachment there is dynamic harmony of affect and intention, a kind of interactive synchrony. During a phase of alert engagement, the interaction of mothers with their infants has been likened to a dance, in which affective signals and moves of the dance are sequential, reciprocal, and contingent such that they manifest a harmony of emotion and intention [13–15]. Critical to secure attachment and the child's self-esteem is thus infant–mother coordination of communication in the moment, and the capacity for "affective reparation" [16].

Emotional self-regulation can be viewed as a related theme of development, which depends upon security of attachment. In marching toward greater proficiency in independent behavior, the growing child must master reflexive, potentially excessive emotional response to frustration in order to favor reflexive, more advanced cognitive and communicative strategies. Whereas the infant internalizes an image of a rescuing parent at moments of distress, the toddler will hopefully have an inner model of this rescue which fosters self-soothing, which in turn allows for a pause to consider a range of options (which might however involve calling out for the parent). In a review of emotion regulation, Cassidy and Berlin [17] illustrate that the empathic parent provides for, not only a soothing and dampening down of negative emotion, but also direct encouragement of positive affective states. Thus, in addition to their role in unconscious attunement to the child's affect, parents consciously correct and socialize the child's response to frustration, generally by providing examples and explicit advice.

To further clarify the role of attachment in emotion regulation, reference should be made to the psychological principle of "scaffolding," a term coined by Vygotsky [18]. According to this principal, an available and caring adult interprets the child's interest and capacity, and with this reference in mind will aid the child in advancing to a new level, either in learning a task or with a method of coping with challenge. We may conclude that "good enough" attachment works at the child's "proximal zone of development," and involves both a shared emotional and shared cognitive frame of reference in an ongoing, dynamic process which is normally strengthened by ties of affection.

Definition of Reactive Attachment Disorder (RAD)

According to DSM-IV the essential feature of RAD is marked disturbance of social relatedness in most contexts that begins before age 5, and which is preceded by grossly pathogenic care [19]. Children with RAD may present in two quite different, even opposite-appearing subtypes: those who withdraw from interpersonal encounter, RAD inhibited-withdrawn type; and the RAD disinhibited-indiscriminate type, those who show little reserve toward strangers and seem impulsive as well as nonselective in the pattern of relationship. Key to both types of attachment disorder is absence of selective proximity-seeking: the child does not go to the familiar caregiver in time of distress and, thus, does not appear to use this person as a safe "home base" from which to explore outward. Children with the disinhibited form may literally meet strangers with open arms, thus appearing to devalue the special relationship with a parent figure (and often worrying them on the matter of safety in public). In contrast, children with the withdrawn, inhibited subtype are reluctant to engage with their parent figure, or they might comply mechanically and without feeling. Reunions after time apart may be emotionally charged but ambivalent; the child pulls away or avoids eye contact, which may shake the caregiver's faith in the possibility for growth in the fragile, nascent attachment.

Differential Diagnosis

The historic pattern of symptoms is critical in distinguishing RAD from other childhood disorders, including childhood post-traumatic stress disorder (PTSD) and autism spectrum disorders (ASD). The criterion of severe pathological neglect for RAD seems clear enough; however, we face a practical problem when – as often occurs – records are lost in a transfer between the time of removal from the original home and a foster placement. Can the effects of the early environment be surmised from impressions of case managers who have only recently taken up the case? The child's own history is necessarily limited: pathogenic care will often have occurred prior to their use of words to describe the environment or their responses to it. Frequent shifts of many children with RAD in the foster care system paradoxically shifts the responsibility for history onto the new adult caregivers, even when they have only brief acquaintance with the child [20]. Reliability of diagnosis can, of course be improved by direct observation of the children interacting with their caregivers. Clinical scales may also usefully supplement the child psychiatry assessment and can help direct investigation of identified problem areas [21].

In the real-time clinic interview, children with the inhibited withdrawn form of RAD may resemble children with ASD in level of emotional detachment, and lack of reciprocity. Rutter et al. [22] studied children with early, severe deprivation and described "quasi-autistic features" which included lack of social awareness and lack of observance of personal boundaries. Both types of RAD however separate from ASD in the longitudinal pattern course of symptoms. RAD children may show social inhibition, but eventually are congruent and reciprocal in the use of nonverbal and verbal communication with their parent figure. Other signs of ASD such as repetitive stereotyped behavior and restricted range of interest are also absent in RAD. Language delay is commonly present in RAD at time of placement removal from an adverse setting, but progressively improves, unlike the case of ASD. Children with RAD do not demonstrate the idiosyncratic language of ASD, such as echolalia or pronoun reversal.

Because of the effect of early childhood maltreatment on language, the diagnosis of mixed receptive-expressive language delay must also be distinguished from RAD based on symptom course. In RAD, language including its pragmatic elements is available as "equipment" for attachment, yet is not applied normally to enhance a selective interpersonal bond. Verbal expression of emotion may lag behind the generally positive course for language development in children removed from adverse environments (see section Alexithymia to follow).

Given the impact of gross pathogenic care in early childhood, it is often difficult to distinguish symptoms of RAD from those of PTSD. A practical question is whether the clinician can reasonably differentiate post-traumatic symptoms from those of attachment disorder. Hyper-arousal and hyper-vigilance could certainly compromise the capacity for trust in attachment for children with PTSD. A distinguishing feature of RAD is, however, the worsening of behavioral symptoms as familiarity increases with the new caregivers, as if progressive intimacy presented a new stress, rather than a reassurance. Though not a formal diagnostic criterion, this tendency to worsen under conditions of environmental constancy can be a "hard sign" for RAD. The child's history – when reliably obtained – is the most determining of diagnosis: in PTSD there is one or more instances of trauma which produce symptoms, whereas for RAD there is early deprivation followed by impairment in progressive attachment to the parent figures, as well as by general impairment in social relations.

Comorbidity

Franc et al. [23] have recently reviewed similarities of RAD with a more common disorder of childhood, attention deficit hyperactivity disorder (ADHD). Although, RAD is rare in comparison to ADHD, there is overlap for some children in the domain of emotional self-regulation – the ability to self-soothe and to organize responses to adverse or challenging stimuli. Intemperate, strongly negative emotional displays often occur in both disorders, sometimes culminating in a trend to oppositional-defiant, disruptive behavior. Conversely, Franc et al. suggest that secure attachment might protect against development of ADHD by promoting cognitive and emotional organization.

Hall and Geher [24] have examined behavioral and personality characteristics of children with RAD. On a broad-range standard symptom inventory, the Child Behavior Checklist [25], children with RAD show both externalizing and internalizing symptoms, including anxiety/depression, thought problems, social problems, and aggressive and delinquent behavior. On other tests, affected children scored low on measures of empathy, and tended to minimize negative personality traits, or to represent them in overly positive ways.

Appropriate assessment of RAD will require multiple encounters, including observations of how the child interacts with familiar caregivers. At the time of initial interview, common comorbid conditions should be considered and identified, including oppositional-defiant symptoms and school adjustment problems [26]. Commercially available surveys which purport to adequately diagnose RAD based upon a composite of comorbidity lack specificity, because of the variability of symptoms within the diagnosis [27]. Routine standard child symptom inventories are recommended instead, for the purpose of identifying comorbidity as well as for prioritizing those interventions which the psychiatrist can provide as a member of the treatment team. Separate forms are available for school-age [25] and for pre-school children [28]. The psychiatrist should be prepared for additional diagnostic assessment of syndromes suggested by the symptom inventory, and for treatment of comorbid conditions including mood and anxiety disorders, PTSD, ADHD, and ODD.

Chapter 2
Vignette of "Jorge"

(A Representative Case for Study)

Part 1: Jorge as a Toddler

Ted and Beth were childless and in their late 30s when they decided to adopt. Beth had postponed pregnancy, determined to earn an advanced degree in linguistics, to build her academic career in foreign languages, and to extend her networking possibilities as a translator. Ted transitioned to a job as an athletics coach after achieving his bachelor's in English literature, not his original aspiration, but rewarding enough in his early career. With local downsizing of the public school, he was compelled to search for new opportunity and eventually landed a job with a landscaping firm. Recently business was slow, but at least the family would not have to move. Over 10 years of marriage without dependents, Ted and Beth were financially secure with their combined salaries and were comfortable with the monthly bills. The Smiths were also happy as a couple, though Beth was aware of Ted's wish for a child and his effort at "not bringing up the subject." Generally they handled the subject with the unwritten rule of "avoiding the subject" or at least maintaining a courteous consideration of each other's feelings. They often reflected that they were lucky as a couple, sharing, for example, their enjoyment of a rural town and many of the same friends from childhood.

Family life changed after the death of Beth's mother, and Ted became consoler and silent support in a winter of extended grieving, during which Beth appeared to lose interest in meeting friends, or even getting out for a walk. Despite the intimacy of a shared or similar experience, their relationship was marked by unaccustomed, minor squabbles, and "arguments over nothing." Beth shared her disappointment in her family of origin; her father and brothers were even more reserved and actually shifted away emotionally despite sharing a loss. It seemed as if with the loss of her mother the family had also lost its center.

Beth and Ted strengthened ties with their church during this period and, possibly influenced by the sight of families with young children, or their new friends, they began to share the idea of a child late in life. Eventually they considered this carefully, even to the extent of meeting with a financial counselor who seemed

D.F. Shreeve, *Reactive Attachment Disorder: A Case-Based Approach*,
SpringerBriefs in Child Development, DOI 10.1007/978-1-4614-1647-0_2,
© Springer Science+Business Media, LLC 2012

determined to temper their zeal with some hard figures. They responded humorously, now sharing an enthusiasm and joy, which seemed to dispel the atmosphere of Beth's winter-long grieving. Beth, now age 39, scheduled a general checkup with their family physician to be sure that neither her age nor any other factor would stop the plan for a child.

An initial, happy anticipation waned as months passed without success in conception. A series of specialists were consulted, for both Ted and Beth, with a full infertility work-up. Gynecology consultation, examinations, and endocrine studies eventually led to diagnosis for Beth of premature ovarian failure. Prognosis was poor for fertility, even with hormone repletion; no treatment was recommended. Beth and Ted faced a new disappointment, turning over together the meaning of such an ironic, and seeming cruel, blow of fate which seemed to test their recent resolve to return to the faith of early childhood. Yet, despite the news, over time they felt stronger in faith and relationship and admonished each other not give in to despairing feelings. It was in the course of their community church activities that, separately and together, they discovered that international adoption appealed to them, based on familiarity with conditions of poverty in many countries, in contrast to their separate and combined economic success in this country.

As required by their private adoption firm, they provided full details about their home, family, and income, and specified only their criteria of a young, healthy child in need of a home. Nevertheless the wait for assignment of a child seemed endless, and after a year their agency informed them that host countries so far contacted had imposed tight restrictions for overseas adoption.

A month later, the Smiths are overjoyed to hear that a further search – extended to Guatemala – had been successful. The boy, Jorge, is "age 3, no evidence of medical problems, mother age 16 not supported." A birth certificate and a certificate of good health can be provided to them through the agency, but there are no pediatric records apart from the medical statement. On request, further records indicate "two previous foster placements", after the orphanage. The Smith's case manager is responsive and wants to help, but admits to frustration reaching the orphanage, or social work authorities in charge of Jorge. Further inquiry results in the information that Jorge's mother was "under age but had no medical problems of concern... and his birth was normal." The case manager is then notified of "additional local fees and costs" necessary to proceed with the adoption. Wanting to have all available information in advance, Beth and Ted press their stateside adoption agency for details, receiving only a terse reply "there is no medical problem, a decision must be made within 4 weeks, not longer." After reflection and a sharing of concerns, the Smiths decide to act: the wait has already gone on too long; they accept assignment of his care, even with the scant available background information.

Beth and Ted have pictures of their new family member, but are taken off guard by their first moments with Jorge: he is much smaller than they had expected for a child nearing his fourth birthday, and he seems much smaller and younger than expected. They reason that Jorge's small size may be within average range in his native region, or close to it. But, even though pre-screening exam listed no abnormalities, his first examination with their family doctor shows him to be below the fifth percentile for both height and weight. The family physician remarks low general muscle tone and asymmetry of lower deep tendon reflexes, as well as poor extensor strength. Bilateral otitis media and end-expiratory wheezing are noted. Jorge's lab reports show mild anemia and leukocytosis with a left shift. There is elevation of serum lead, but not high enough for chelation treatment. Chest x-ray is read as normal. Needed vaccinations are scheduled. The Smith's family physician recommends further consultation with pediatrics, and a "full developmental assessment."

Case Point: International Adoption

It may be reasonably asked why a couple as determined and organized as the Smiths would not have demanded and received full medical information on Jorge. Recent televised and written documentaries by John Seabrook [29, 30] highlight the risks and benefits, as well as complexities of international adoptive process. Briefly summarized, a "global migration" of orphan children to the USA began in China, Vietnam, and Korea in the 1950s and then shifted to involve primarily Latin American and Eastern Europe by the end of the 1980s. More than 226,000 children were internationally adopted into the USA between 1990 and 2005 [31].

A reasonable argument favoring international adoption, as Seabrook points out is that "poorer nations have much higher birth rates and so there is a global imbalance in children and the resources needed to raise them out of poverty" [29]. Countries with children who need homes follow a similar political path, however. According to Seabrook, "a nation opens its borders, adoptions proliferate; corruption creeps in; there is a scandal, the borders close." A Guatemalan example is depicted by Dubinsky [32]; a kidnapping of a child led to rumors of widespread trafficking in children. The rumors were evidently fueled by public sentiment about the many homeless plainly visible on the street, a sight which can inspire a kind of national shame and then culminating in restrictions on the adoption process. Similarly, Kim [33] reports that the Seoul International Olympics in 1988 attracted public interest in Korean culture, and this in turn inspired news reports which included the April 21 1988 *New York Times* article on "Babies for Export," a report which hurt Korean pride and eventually led to "systematic discouragement of international adoption" and thus to the target of zero adoptions to the USA.

The global need for stable adoptive homes continues to increase even as political factors – including the policing of human trafficking – have greatly reduced access for international adoption. UNICEF recently estimated the number of children worldwide who need homes at 163 million [29]. Yet the rate of adoptions into the USA has plummeted, from its peak in 2004 of 22,884 (from more than 90 nations) to a figure less than half this number. According to Seabrook, "the process is dwindling because no one can agree on what constitutes an ethical adoption."

During the wave of international adoption that ended in 2004, the mix of adoptees shifted dramatically from 37% Korean in 1990 with 3% Eastern Europe to 65%

Eastern Europe and just 10% Korean by 2000 [31]. This variable "country of origin" crucially affects the study of attachment because of the superior care of orphans generally provided in Korea, where foster care is in the hands of state-trained and monitored foster guardians [31, 33]. This is to compare to the care received in the notorious state-run orphanages of Romania during the Ceausescu regime, a context that is clearly associated with attachment disorder in childhood [34].

Nowadays few adoptees from overseas are "war orphans" and most have been abandoned, or given up because of poverty. Parents in the USA who seek to adopt from another country have limited ability to require particular attributes, due to diminishing numbers of children available from their country of origin. Conditions of health status can be specified, but the power to enforce these conditions is limited. Affecting this phenomenon of supply and demand is the parallel stateside adoptive process: the number of healthy infants in the USA available for adoption has also sharply declined, at least for young children not previously adopted and without special needs. Factors which influence this supply include the impact of birth control and the rise of single parenting. Most of the domestic adoptions are now relatively older children, as compared to 10 years ago, and many come from foster care.

Part 2: Jorge at Preschool Age

The Smiths are quick to set up an appointment in the nearby university Developmental Pediatric Clinic. Examinations confirm the prior findings of poor general muscle tone and poor upper and lower extensor strength. Also noted is restricted left wrist range of motion and poor balance on either leg. On careful exam, Jorge has a swinging of the left gain on ambulation, so that he has a limp, more pronounced when he attempts to ambulate rapidly. The remainder of the examination, including cardiac auscultation and pulmonary exam, is unremarkable. With help from an interpreter, the team is able to complete a range of developmental tests, leading to the conclusion that Jorge shows general delay in adaptive skills including hygiene and self-dressing. In addition to annotating these multiple delays, the team lists diagnosis of "probable attention deficit hyperactivity disorder" and "rule out neglect and/or physical abuse in early life." Based on the observable limp, and wrist contracture, full skeletal series is recommended. Subsequent radiology results include the report of, "focal bony irregularity along the distal right tibia suggests prior remote trauma." Jorge is scheduled with physical therapy for work on balance, ambulation, and upper extremity range of motion remediation therapy. Although psychiatry consultation is also recommended at this point, the Smiths defer on this last point, emphasizing their hope that behavioral symptoms will respond to "kindness and consistency in a good home."

In the initial experience with Jorge, the Smiths feel confirmed about their choices in the treatment plan, and in their hopes for Jorge. Despite some physical delays, Jorge shows boundless energy and is very active in exploring his new environment.

He is "in constant motion," and the effort to track him is greater than the Smith's had anticipated. Mild clumsiness for age and frequent falls also do not discourage him from exploring every nook and cranny of the new home. At times he will run straight into their arms and, forcefully, a little too fast for comfort. His adoptive parents are impressed by his affection toward them and toward adult friends who visit, but begin to worry about his safety in public. Increasingly, they share their worry about his safety with strangers. They find comfort in the advice that Jorge is "making up for lost time," perhaps compensating for early life deprivation and hearing problems, the latter possibly affecting delay of language. Privately they share their misgivings however, and guilt about their resentment of Jorge's nonselective display of affection. They are relieved by the school recommendation to delay Jorge a year before kindergarten; this is based on the hope that he will catch up with children of his grade level in size, while advancing in a new language. Beth and Ted agree with this, but would like to put off evaluation by child psychiatry, or further psychology testing, because they are confident that "everything can improve with enough time and love."

Case Point: Neglect, Growth, and Medical Problems

The finding of small body size in orphan children led to the theory that supports the idea that emotional deprivation directly retards growth, perhaps mediated by stress effects on the hypothalamic-pituitary-adrenal (HPA) axis. The evaluation of Failure to Thrive (FTN) is complex, however, because of frequent overlap of emotional deprivation, malnutrition, and stress in the affected families [35]. The hypothesis that emotional neglect has a direct biological effect on growth is challenged by studies showing at least a partial compensation in growth rate after provision of a fully adequate diet [36]. Stunting of growth and deficits of attachment are now recognized as separate effects of severe early childhood deprivation [37].

With regard to our case "Jorge," the Guatemalan record is certainly benign in comparison to the costs of the Ceausescu regime to orphan children. Miller et al. [38] have assessed the children adopted from Guatemala into the USA, for comparison to US norms in case-matched design study. A growth delay is commonly found at adoption, and is generally more severe for children from Guatemalan orphanages as compared to Guatemalan children adopted from foster care. Children adopted at young age improved most quickly in their new stateside homes. The authors also report the large number of children involved: more than 17,300 in the period of 1986–2005. In addition to growth delays in height, weight, and head circumference, the children had relatively high rates of anemia (30%) and elevated serum lead levels (3%), as well as high rate for latent tuberculosis (7%). Only 28% met American Academy of Pediatrics standards for vaccine administration.

For adopted children with FTN, there is good reason to be hopeful about the trajectory toward normal physical growth in a new adoptive home that provides appropriate nutrition. In comparison, relatively more caution applies to questions from adoptive parents about the prospect for full emotional recovery from early deprivation, neglect, or abuse. Grossly pathogenic care at critical stages of early childhood raises the risk for childhood disorders which are comorbid with RAD, including disruptive behavior disorders, post-traumatic stress disorder, depression, and anxiety [39, 40]. Counseling a family about relative risk for these conditions can help families prepare for challenges ahead, and this can be a helpful intervention even at early points of mental health assessment.

Part 3: Jorge in Kindergarten

During the time Jorge delayed from starting kindergarten, Ted and Beth have wasted no time in aligning developmental services, to include physical therapy, occupational therapy, and home tutoring. Beth is pleased to have a new use for her love of languages, and Jorge responds warmly to her Spanish. Many evenings, the two play on the rug with toys, or share picture books, English to Spanish and Spanish to English. Ted enjoys the family scene but admits half-jokingly to a feeling of exclusion: Jorge seems oblivious to his efforts at beginning Spanish. He will sometimes reply in English, but the Smiths consult a speech and language therapist about a new symptom: sometimes Jorge will not respond to either of them, in either language. With further analysis, the selective inattention is found to be related to a developing opposition to rules, such as bed times, or anything interrupting play. To curb his new, facultative, language problem, Beth is encouraged to stop trying in Spanish, and both adoptive parents are to give simple explanations of expectations in English, employing eye contact and, if necessary, applying a "consequence" (such as removal of a toy for a time) when Jorge postpones compliance.

Optimism at home is also tempered by Jorge's behavior in public. At church he is more hyperactive, and sometimes frankly disregards instructions to stay with them, or to stay quiet. He is also too forward with strangers, abruptly giving a hug at unpredictable moments or, for example, taking the hand of an adult as if going for a walk with a complete stranger. They see the same problem at a restaurant or going to a movie; Jorge now seems uninhibited about starting conversation in English with adults unknown to the Smith household. His capacity to verbalize, and even use colloquial American speech, is remarkable, but Beth especially is hurt by the comparison to the rudimentary conversation which can be supported at home.

The start of kindergarten greatly magnifies and expands Jorge's difficulty with social distance: his teacher is quick to identify a problem with "getting too close" with children he has not met, and parents have closely questioned Beth and Ted on this. Sometimes he runs directly into a child with arms open, in something like a hug, but he sometimes slaps the arm or head too roughly, so that the meaning of the gesture seems midway between expressing hostility or inviting friendship. Both parents have researched the library and the web for age-appropriate materials to teach Jorge about "stranger danger" and "good touch bad touch." Results are inconclusive, though he seems to listen and attend to their gentle efforts.

Meanwhile Jorge is alternatively argumentative or over-affectionate with same-age children who Beth and Ted invite over for playmates: Jorge will sometimes share his toys but can become suddenly pushy and aggressive; his new friends tell their parents they do not wish to return because "he's too bossy."

Jorge does not show expected improvement in his early weeks of kindergarten but seems to grow steadily worse in offending other children and in refusal to sit in a circle or share in games. There is question about his earlier progress in English language comprehension, and he seldom replies directly to the teacher. Beth and Ted this time agree to both psychology and psychiatry consultations, as suggested by the school.

At first appointment with Jorge and his family, Ted and Beth share their chief concerns as Jorge looks on silently, and he declines to join in discussion at this point, even with gentle support. Chief complaints thus are from the parents: (1) a growing pattern of intermittent, unguarded intimacy with adults, such as importune advance and start of conversation with complete strangers, and (2) irritability and apparent hostility toward them, especially when Jorge is asked to interrupt play, to get ready for bed, or to prepare for school. What stands out from the next individual interview with Jorge is his free use of language and his casual and apparently friendly behavior. He quickly finds toy puppets and seems familiar with how to use puppets to represent a pretend conversation. He will converse freely with this device and seems to enjoy new acquaintance, smiling warmly even in his first session. Jorge falls silent however, in the face of questions about his early home, and is finally mute when problems in his life with Ted and Beth are gently approached.

Another remarkable feature of the combined interviews is Jorge's lack of emotional expression or protest when his parents go to the waiting room to allow individual work. They try to prepare him for a possible distressing shift, but he seems too busy with toys to care at this point. Even more startling, there is no visible shift in expression, and no verbal acknowledgement of their return, at the time of reunion for discussion of preliminary findings. These are discussed with the Smiths in terms of a preliminary, differential diagnosis based on symptoms including hyperactivity and also on the history of presumed trauma and multiple placements. Attention Deficit Hyperactivity Disorder (ADHD), PTSD, and RAD are each explained in terms of understanding. In addition, the autistic spectrum disorders are reviewed as a rule out, with the caveat that Jorge has certainly shown a full range of nonverbal expression, has made progress in language, and at least sometimes will share a fun activity interactively. ADHD symptom checklists are provided to survey symptoms at home and school. The Child Behavior Checklist is to be completed at home and returned. Referral to a psychology colleague is also made at this point, for impressions on the differential diagnosis, and for further tests of aptitude and development.

Findings from psychology consultation specifically do not support Autistic Spectrum Disorder (ASD). On an observation-based diagnostic instrument, the Child Autistic Rating Scale [41], Jorge's scores are in the nonclinical range. The report also lists Jorge's eagerness to relate to the examiner, his reciprocal style of play behavior in the exam room, and his open expression of pleasure with the social encounter.

Also noted is the recent, remarkable advance in language, which does not seem consistent with autistic spectrum. His skillful use of facial expression and nonverbal expressiveness is also remarked. Further developmental evaluation was recommended, especially to follow the direction of learning disorder, possible improvement in language, and to rule out attachment disorder. Close pediatric care is encouraged, with the range of medical findings already identified. Jorge's social disadvantage with peers is remarked, based on his small body size. Psychology suggests that a portion of his oppositional behavior at home, and also his preference for adult company might relate to negative self-attributions and comparisons about body size, his limp, and his sense of cultural distance from peers.

Consult to orthopedics for evaluation of a limp and wrist has led to extensive evaluation of boney defects and in turn to medical evaluations which have ruled out pediatric congenital bone disease. Uneven leg length is considered a factor in the limp. Foot x-rays however reveal "metatarsal distal flaring, possibly due to early metaphysis tearing and callous reformation." No treatment is recommended except for the limp, a condition that is now obviously a problem when Jorge tries to join in play with other children when this involves running or moving rapidly. Beth brings Jorge back to his physical therapy, but he says he does not remember her and becomes immediately angry in the clinic, folding his arms and refusing to move from the waiting room. Report from the session is that he is now "too hyperactive and disruptive to engage in treatment." Beth and Ted now have a physical therapy regimen to try at home with Jorge, in hopes of improving his balance and gait. Since the family continues to decline to consider psychotropic medications, they elect to follow-up in 3 months, with the offer to come in earlier if symptoms require.

Case Point: The Retrospective Evaluation of Child Abuse

The child psychiatry clinician and radiologist seem to rarely share cases, but one example share of partnership involves the difficult assessment of infant abuse when evaluation takes place years later, as might occur in the case of international adoption. In such a case, past medical records are sparse, even missing. But even more fundamental is a special quality of the infant skeleton: it is amazingly flexible, and this, with the restructuring of growing bone, makes diagnosis by plane film especially problematic. Isolated fractures may heal in place, without a residual change in contour. Rib fractures (a common sign of severe infant trauma), for example, may be invisible years after injury.

Other reliable signs of child abuse which are familiar to emergency room clinicians are likewise less dependable when injury occurs in infancy. Cigarette burns may have healed, or morphed into vague skin discolorations. The clinical sign "wounds of different ages" will not apply assuming the child has not had subsequent, serial trauma after removal from the original setting of abuse. Displaced fractures sometimes may heal in nonalignment, however, and would then be visible on x-ray. An unfortunate example occurs when an adult, in the act of changing diapers, becomes enraged and twists forcefully on both femoral bones; an injury of this kind could plausibly cause a limp for a child like in our case of Jorge, and could be discoverable years after injury [42]. Assaults on infants typically injure long bones and the feet are spared [43]. An exception is a grabbing and yanking injury to the feet, and severe foot fractures almost invariably involve metatarsal bones.

Physical abuse of infants may also cause bowing of either femur or tibia bones, and the fracture line may be invisible on plane film [44]. The powerful force that can produce such trauma transmits itself to the ends of long bones, with a valvular deformation at the proximal tibia, or with fracture to the growth plate. One telltale sign is called the "classic metaphyseal lesion" [44] and this is a fracture through the growth plate, best viewed with photomicrography. As the fracture spreads laterally, it flares out and separates the bony collar underlying the periosteum from the cortex of bone. With angular beaming technology, the end of the long bone may show a "bucket handle" shape, which indicates the early trauma of impact to the long bone, manifest at the "weak spot" of the growth plate. In addition to bone injuries in infancy, tendon burn injuries are an additional cause for a residual limp, as in the case of Jorge [42].

Late interpretation of infant abuse is an art as well as a science, and is rarely considered in part because it will not lead to information that guides any new medical treatment. It is also true that few children with multiple severe injuries of this kind actually survive: head trauma in combination with rib fracture, for example, is typically fatal [45]. Given the limitations of a purely medical assessment, the findings of child mental health will carry considerable weight in the interpretation of early trauma. The child psychiatry equivalent for "wounds of different ages" may be the description of post-traumatic stress disorder which is age specific in its expression and measurable by comparison to norms for age and level of development. Early trauma impacts upon multiple developmental domains, beginning with a lesion to basic trust and expanding to involve delays in emotion regulation, intellectual growth, and social relationship.

Part 4: Jorge in First Grade

Through kindergarten Jorge has gained weight quickly. There is marked improvement in expressive language, a proof for the work of his special education tutor. Now in first grade, he is roughly the same size as other children. He resembles the other children at casual glance, except that he does not share in games and often interferes when other children play together. He cannot relax his exclusive claim to his teacher, and will try to block any other child who tries to approach her. When called upon to explain himself to her, he smiles winningly, and moves closer to her side. Recently, Jorge has shown greater persistence in his effort to sit in his teacher's lap while she is telling a story to the class, and she is increasingly uncomfortable with this behavior. In parallel with his display of affection toward the teacher, he is increasingly aggressive toward his classmates; he has been chastised for "accidentally" kicking or tripping. Most worrisome is the increasing purposefulness of his actions, for which he offers little explanation. He is in fact silent in the face of a scolding and correction, and at time he is mute in class for no apparent cause, disregarding his teacher or others when they try to gain his attention. He also maintains a grudge, and will retaliate long after an argument. Punishment by "time out" is uniformly followed by aggressive behavior, usually a fight with another child. He has had one out of school suspension of a week, for "damage to school property, verbal aggression and out of control behavior."

Jorge is by now assigned to a counselor at school, who is trying to understand the causes for his unpredictable hostility, while at the same time coaching him in social skills. Her preliminary impression is that Jorge has advanced in general English language skills, but lacks a sense of how to label his own emotions, and is misunderstanding the nonverbal, contextual cues he needs to comprehend the group around him. He does not, for example, easily comprehend the difference between "getting mad" as an emotional experience and actually being aggressive as in hurting another child or damaging property. He blandly denies both anger and angry behavior, at first not understanding a clear distinction. His therapist discovers that when Jorge plays a competitive game with the other first graders, he perceives them to be cheating, even conspiring together if he does not win. He is thus inclined to label laughter of a child as "laughing at him." He also explains his problem behaviors, such as tripping or hitting other children, as necessary to maintaining his social standing with his peers, and in fact he feels those that provoke or test him are personally responsible for his violence. Counseling is now directed to both decoding and reframing the meaning of his arguments with other children, and there is consideration of expanding to a social skills group, to try out his new ideas about how to relate to children and teachers in the classroom.

Case Point: Alexythymia and Attachment

In addition to its instrumental goal of exchanging information, first use of words is profoundly personal, and in the early dyadic relationship it comprises an extension of the principle of attunement to the moment of shared experience. The relationship of language to attachment seems certain, based on empiric research; an example is the finding that the hormone oxytocin – which mediates human attachment behavior – increases when young girls (age 7–12) are comforted by the voice of their own mother, during a stress test which requires timed mathematical tasks in front of an audience [46]. Conversely, selective mutism may reveal deficits of child attachment, or may reflect the child's perception of adult misattunement [47]. It is therefore encouraging to witness the rapid, and sometimes amazing, advance in the use of language for a child with RAD, after their transfer from conditions of emotional deprivation to a new, supportive home.

Capacity for selective attachment lags behind the general advance in language after transfer to a new home. This introduces the question of whether use of language to express personal emotion might be a specific impairment. Development of emotions-related language can be studied in children through analysis of social measures, and scales of social competence have been applied to research on RAD [48]. Alexithymia is the term, first coined by Sifneos [49], for an evident deficit in symbolization of somatic and mental states (he applied the term to adult patients with psychosomatic disorders). In their study of alexithymia in children, Way et al. [50] redefine alexithymia as "cognitive-affective communication impairment" and a "psychological phenomenon in which individuals may experience or be aware of strong feelings but have difficulty understanding and effectively expressing their feelings to others." They apply the term to a child who cannot identify their subjective experience of emotion and, hence, cannot convey the experience to others.

Externalizing symptoms, especially aggression, frequently correlate with impoverishment of language skills. On this basis, Way et al. [50] propose a fundamental relationship between childhood problems in communication, and delay in emotional self-regulation. Language disability is thus one element of the differential diagnosis of childhood aggression: outbursts of violence in a child may represent in part, a disability in communicating emotion by other means. Conversely, a child with language delay is at risk for academic and social problems. Of particular importance is the expressive deficit which may be specifically targeted in school even as a comorbid receptive language delay – perhaps less obvious but equally telling – continues to bar the way to normal relationship. Mixed delays are the rule rather than the exception, and many children with externalizing symptoms do not comprehend, or at least do not use nonverbal, pragmatic language cues to efficiently coordinate social intercourse. Inaccuracies in interpretation predispose to social ostracism, can lead to negative self-attributions, and hence may facilitate further use of "acting out" as the default method for expression of negative emotion [51].

The relationship between social development and use of emotional language is complex because the use of emotion words also requires motivation for emotional language and, in this sense, a matrix of attachment. Zadeh et al. [52] propose a model for language as a mediating influence between social cognition and psychopathology in externalizing children: the effective use of positive social strategies requires skillful use of language (especially syntax) because of the importance of taking perspective (representing perspective of oneself and another). These results support a dual approach to externalizing children, emphasizing both language competence and social-cognitive therapy.

Lemche et al. [48] have directly measured alexithymia in children with different levels, or subtypes of attachment. The authors assigned infants in the study at 12 months using the Strange Situation, into the categories of secure and insecure subtypes. Subsequently, at age 17, 23, 30, and 36 months, transcripts of the children's language were collected under controlled conditions. Significant differences emerge between secure and insecure children: insecure avoidant and insecure disorganized toddlers show marked delay in use of words to express inner state of emotion, a meager vocabulary for words which pertain to emotional regulation, and rare use of words to represent internal physiological states (e.g., "thirsty"). Children classified as secure infants were more likely at 17 months to use "positive emotion words," in addition to using more words to self-regulate, or to depict physiological state. The measures of alexithymia persist in the insecure children, as late as 3 years into the study. The authors thus conclude that attachment status in infancy predicts the trajectory of a childhood capacity to symbolize and manage emotion.

Pivotal to our study of language and attachment is the effect of infant maltreatment on subsequent emotional expression. In an abusive or neglectful home, the young child is primarily exposed to negative affect, and receives few confirmations of positive, reciprocal communications either verbal or nonverbal. Camras et al. [53] explored the effect of maternal facial expressivity in a comparison of 20 maltreated with 20 non-maltreated children. Facial expressivity of the children was essentially proportional to maternal expressivity, for both groups. In general, children of mothers with high facial expressivity were better at interpreting emotion. Older children also scored higher than younger children. But the key finding is the consistently higher scores in emotional recognition for non-maltreated control children, for emotions ranging from pure happiness through sadness, fear, surprise, and disgust. When cognitive maturity is factored out (using the Peabody Picture Vocabulary Test), the finding holds true that maltreatment status conveys a disadvantage in accurately recognizing the emotional content of facial expressions.

Germane to a consideration of emotional intelligence in attachment-disordered children is the analysis by Wismer Fries and Pollak [54] of affect recognition abilities of post-institutionalized Eastern European children. The study group had resided in orphanages for an average of 16.6 months prior to adoption. For the 18 post-institutional children a significant handicap was discovered, in comparison to controls in interpreting test faces depicting emotion, as well as in matching standard facial expressions with emotional situation in quantitative measures of emotion discrimination.

The evidence for impoverishment of emotion recognition as a function of early emotional deprivation points to an expanded role of speech and language pathology, which is based on dyadic relationship of early life. Geller and Foley [55] advocate for expansion of the field of speech pathology to incorporate advances in the understanding of the emotional foundation for use of language in early childhood. Essentially the model involves "working from the inside out"; the authors explain that language deficits may be formulated in terms of parental understanding of the child, their hopes and wishes, as well as the child's own state of affect and need to communicate. Geller and Foley emphasize the importance of attachment theory, and the understanding of past and present relationship of parent and child. For this expanding role of speech and language pathology, the authors emphasize applications for Stern's theory of emotional attunement and encourage the clinician's therapeutic use of the "self" in treatment.

Part 5: Jorge in Second and Third Grades

As the treating child psychiatrist you are invited to participate in an Individualized Education Plan for second Grade. Parents and school are united in their concern about Jorge's disruptive behavior, his poor peer relationships, and by his apparent insatiable hunger for adult attention. There is overt encouragement to consider medication treatment for hyperactivity. In addition to this consideration, his new education plan will include full in-school assignment of a teacher's aide. In addition to providing an adult emotional support, the aide will view and supervise relationship with other children, to encourage a pro-social trend. In addition, a new element of the education plan is "time in" for Jorge, a period of close, individual attention away from the other children and with his teacher's aide, after each incident of unruly behavior. This contingent response is intended to reverse the effect of rejection that seems implicit in the "time out" which has been used as a consequence for problem behavior.

The new plan meets with initial success; Jorge and his assigned aide seem to warm toward each other quickly, and he responds to her directions at first. But this impression shifts as he begins to test her authority, while simultaneously "demanding hugs all through the class." Adults share their dismay about a new behavior of "combined hugs and hits"; Jorge will come running into the arms of his teacher or his aide, and the forceful lunge feels hostile, even deliberately hurtful. Jorge only smiles when the effect is questioned, so that the question remains as to whether he intends to be aggressive or whether he is perhaps clumsy, even off balance because of his limp.

Medication treatment for hyperactivity in the final semester of second grade also has a hopeful beginning, and Jorge shows initial rapid improvement in listening skills, with a modest enhancement of sharing with other children. There is brief cessation of the "running hugs" of adults (hug combined with collision), which had offended several of the teachers. Report for parent–teacher conference includes the optimistic finding that "Jorge exhibits a degree of calm he has never shown before."

Success is short lived, and a new problem behavior emerges: from an initial warming of affection toward his teacher's aide, Jorge is now pressing her continuously for physical affection, and continuous, exclusive attention. After an eerie episode in which Jorge tries to kiss and stroke her arms, his teacher's aide threatens to quit, and the plan to assign an adult to Jorge in his half day of mainstream class is abandoned. Without this resource, Jorge's aggression toward other children rapidly worsens, leading to a theory of some in school that he is deliberately retaliating. Jorge is often in trouble during recess for tripping other children, a behavior he denies with a smile, but one that has been witnessed, then documented. He finally receives an out-of-school suspension for allegedly stabbing a child in the face with a pencil, during an argument at lunchtime. Jorge explains this as accidental, and though the injury is superficial, the school is under pressure from the parent of the injured child to take action.

Based on mixed or unclear results, you elect to suspend the medication treatment during summer, and you schedule reevaluation before the start of third grade. It is at this point that the parents divide in their approach to treatment. His mother would like to continue psychiatry appointments but to "try something different." His father has become interested in a form of attachment therapy which, per description of Jorge's parents, advocates strict discipline "twenty-four seven," recommends use of "forced holds" and opposes all forms of psychiatry treatment. Ted explains to you his opinion that RAD is "not biological and not medical" and that he adds that he has learned on a web site that "symptoms get worse on a medication through kindling." Following a discussion between Jorge's parents at home, his mother calls to suspend appointments, she confides that marital problems have recently complicated life at home, to the extent that marital therapy will need to be prioritized, ahead of Jorge's outpatient work for the present.

Case Point: Longitudinal Course and the Trait of Indiscriminate Friendliness

There are few studies for longitudinal course of RAD beyond early childhood. An interesting exception is a long-term study of twins, from 18 months to 8 years [56, 57]. With the effect of ongoing treatment, there was overall clinical improvement for the twins, but residual externalizing symptoms. Persistence of self-endangering behaviors suggests the early, traumatic effect of pathogenic care in this case study.

Longitudinal studies reveal persistence of attachment disorder symptoms after adoption, for children initially abandoned and then raised in a residential nursery in which personal contact was minimized, but physical stimuli – books and toys – were provided [58, 59]. Of 26 children who remained institutionalized for the first 4 years of life, eight were identified as emotionally withdrawn and unresponsive, ten were indiscriminately social, and eight were selective in attachment to their caregiver. The "over-friendly" attention-seeking trait was found to be especially persistent for these post-institutional children as observed at 4–8 years. By age 16, indiscriminate behavior toward adults was eclipsed by a related problem of superficiality toward peers, and the affected children appeared to confuse acquaintance with the terms of close friendship [60].

Large-scale studies confirm the impression that, despite the dramatic appearance of the withdrawn-inhibited form of RAD at time of diagnosis, it is the indiscriminate-disinhibited type that shows greater resistance to change after removal from pathogenic care. Social disinhibition persists, for example, in an open lack of reserve toward novel acquaintances and in "wandering off with strangers." In the large-scale English and Romanian Adoption Study, indiscriminate sociability and disinhibition persisted from age 6 to age 11 [61]. Chisholm [62] also reports stability in Romanian orphans for the trait of indiscriminate social behavior, a clinical marker now termed "indiscriminate friendliness."

Indiscriminate friendliness (IF) has been measured for relationship to other clinical syndromes, especially those involving externalizing disorder. Lyons-Ruth et al. [63] used the Strange Situation test to code IF behavior; children who were highly indiscriminate at 18 months also scored high on teachers rating of hyperactivity at kindergarten, independent of the effect of disorganized and avoidant attachment at the same point. Outcome studies of preschool children [60, 64, 65] and school-age children [59] suggest a moderate, inverse relationship of the "over-friendly" (IF) trait with measures of inhibitory control.

Effect of early adverse environment on the trait of indiscriminate sociability has also been examined, independent of the diagnosis of attachment disorder. Bruce et al. [31] have studied a group of 120 children age 6–7 adopted into the USA after receiving institutional or adoptive care for "most of their lives." The authors discovered that adoptees from foreign institutional settings had relatively high levels of IF, but surprisingly this trait was also represented in international adoptees from foster care settings. The institutional care group scored relatively poorly on tests of basic emotional abilities (including tests for recognition of faces depicting emotions) and inhibitory control (including tests to inhibit reflexive response to stimuli). Based on parent reports, disinhibited social behavior was related to the duration but not the degree of general deprivation. For the children from previous institutional care, the level of disinhibited social behavior correlated with length in institutional care, prior to adoption.

In a US study, Pears et al. [64] report a direct relationship between maltreatment and level of IF in foster care children. Children with the highest number of foster care placements showed the poorest level of inhibitory control, and the highest level of IF, leading to an hypothesis for relationship of these variables to a "larger pattern of dysregulation associated with inconsistency in caregiving."

A common finding for each outcome of the study is that disinhibited social behavior specifically corresponds to lack of consistent caregiving in an early, sensitive period of childhood, rather than to general deprivation effects like poor nutrition or lack of medical care [65, 66]. Of note however is the imperfect relationship of the trait of indiscriminate friendliness to nonselective attachment. It is now understood that children raised in institutions may show preference for a particular caregiver, but still display the trait of indiscriminate, disinhibited social behavior [67].

Part 6: Jorge in fourth and fourth Grades

New problems emerge at the start of fourth grade which, from the perspective of involved adults, now eclipse the previous worries about friendship and language delay. These are externalizing symptoms, especially lying, which is pervasive and sometimes oddly without an apparent motive. Pre-meditated or predatory behavior has occurred, such as lying in wait after school to bully smaller children; here lying serves the obvious purpose of denial and minimization. Mistruth about actual homework assignments has complicated his special education plan, and procrastination has evolved into frank opposition to school and schoolwork.

There is also some overlap of distortion with fanciful thinking and even practical jokes. On one occasion, Jorge visited a neighborhood barbecue party and told the adults presiding that Ted and Beth are secretly very poor, to the extent that they are starving him and even "punish him for going in the refrigerator"; this was so convincing that the neighbors prepared him a well-cooked meal. A graver matter is his report to the school guidance counselor that he is often whipped with a belt by his father, and this statement seemed so sincere that a case was filed with Child Protective Services. Jorge has now recanted, but will not explain his motives for the false report.

In the arena of peer relationship, Jorge has yet to find a "best friend." Yet he is often entertaining to a group and has, for example, taught his classmates how to gamble for small coins during recess. At other times he is oddly aloof, and on the playground he sits high up on a slide from which vantage he surveys the other children and the surround, seeming to act like a scout or as if standing guard. On at least one occasion he has baited another child into fighting him, and after the older boy was punished, Jorge confessed to his therapist that bruises and scratches were self-inflicted, a way of "getting him in trouble…and getting him back." This example of self-harm, and the apparent self-defeating behaviors has convinced his therapist that Jorge's best working diagnosis is atypical depression: he is defending against low self-esteem, feelings of rejection, and his earlier self-image as "unloved."

Since release of information is provided, Jorge's therapist is able to communicate her working formulation about Jorge's emerging conduct symptoms: he has not yet achieved sufficient confidence in dyadic relationship to progress to competitive activities with other children, to whom he feels inferior. For the same reason, Jorge rebels against Ted's rule-making, and is jealous of the loving relationship of his adoptive parents. Recommendation is made to Ted to adopt a softer approach, and he agrees to make time each week for positive "fun time" independent of any coaching about rules or school. In addition, both therapist and parents would like opinion about starting an antidepressant medication for Jorge, which hopefully could help his mood, and improve energy available for work and play. A commonly used SSRI is started at low dose, following your review with the family of the current evidence base, and potential risks.

Early effects of this combined approach appear positive. Ted has traded in his sedan for a brand-new off-road vehicle, and has made plans with Jorge for Saturday rides in the country. This is a prized possession for both of them, and part of the day is spent washing and waxing. Ted had to miss one weekend for a business trip, and to his dismay discovers a key or other sharp object has been run across the entire finish. Jorge protests innocence, but Ted will not fully retreat from his accusation that Jorge is somehow responsible, given the unlikelihood of vandalism in their neighborhood, and "based on his lies in the past." According to Beth, Ted now backs away from relationship with Jorge, avoids encounters before school and comes home later in the evening. By report he is opposed both to Jorge's therapy plan, and to future psychiatry appointments.

Following this reversal in relationship Jorge has become more aggressive on the playground. He is more impulsive, for example, walking away from school in plain sight of teachers. Yet he is accused of being more devious: for example putting shards of broken glass in a school mate's shoe, initially denied, and then explained "as a joke." In another apparent effort at a practical joke at home, Jorge pretends to swallow from a bottle of bleach in front of his mother. His simulation of acute illness is so convincing that he is rushed to the emergency room, where he eventually admits his deceit to medical staff, under close questioning. This naturally leads to early psychiatry appointment, and in his next session the SSRI is tapered off, because of correlation with an exacerbation of symptoms.

In the summer after fifth grade, now off medications, frank signs of conduct disorder emerge. Jorge convinces an older boy to jumpstart Ted's off-road vehicle, and the two go joy riding, apprehended only after a minor accident. Following this incident, inventory of mood symptoms is essentially negative, and Jorge has no explanation for the behavior. As the treating child psychiatrist, you again arrange for an early appointment and urge both parents to come for treatment planning. Based on past attendance it is a surprise that the family is a "no-show" to the scheduled session. It is especially unlike Beth not to call to cancel or reschedule. The answer to the mystery arrives as a telephone call from the nearby inpatient child psychiatry hospital; Jorge is an inpatient and his parents would like to arrange follow-up with you after discharge.

The inpatient social worker (with release of information) explains recent symptoms and the need for emergency hospitalization. Prior to admission Jorge elaborated a plan for slowly poisoning Beth, and he posted this on the Internet under the heading "how to murder your mother." In separate sessions he denies the plan, and next explains it as a hoax and a kind of practical joke. Further work on inpatient reveals Jorge's hope that "this will let me get close to my Dad." He seems oblivious of the ramifications of such an action, but seems convincing about his assertion that he "never would really have done it." No other formal thought disorder symptoms were discovered at admission, apart from this remarkable impairment of insight.

Provisional diagnosis from inpatient is bipolar disorder, mixed. This is based on past reckless impulsivity, the possible activation by an antidepressant earlier, and the elaborate homicidal fantasy. A neuroleptic medication has been started at low dose as a mood stabilizer, and after a few days a new antidepressant agent has been started, after psychological assessment, and the finding of an elevation of the depression scale on one of the tests used.

The inpatient record mentions that Jorge never requested calls to his family, as was his privilege. He was calm and agreeable in early family work and in fact seemed to "act as if nothing happened" according to case notes. An early inpatient problem was his frequent request for snacks, and his habit of "hanging out" at the nurse's station. A portion of the inpatient staff supported frequent snack is a necessary comfort for Jorge, helping him cope with emotions during high stress periods such as before group therapy. Others argued that acquiescing to comfort eating has supported a dysfunctional demand to "always get his own way." The complicating problem is weight gain, and even before starting medications on inpatient, the scales show Jorge to be overweight for his age and especially for his height. Weight gain on inpatient is remarkable. Jorge has assaulted another teenager who called him "fatty" and attempted to fight with another boy who imitated him. Jorge has been restrained on inpatient after striking a staff member who tried to control his aggression. The inpatient social worker who is setting up services with you confides that he "was getting worse the longer he stays here"

Test #1: Case-Related Questions

1. Suppose you are the first US physician to meet with Jorge, immediately following his move to a new home with Beth and Ted. At his appointment his case manager tells you that she is concerned about Jorge's growth rate and he appears small for age. She has brought paperwork which includes a brief, hand-written physical examination with the remark "below the fifth percentile for height and weight. Ted and Beth are in attendance too, and add the remark that Jorge is "constantly on the go," very restless physically. Choose the best recommendation based on these initial concerns and the information provided:
   (a) Since small body size is likely to impair self-esteem and impede normal development of friendship, a hormonal treatment to promote rapid growth and weight gain should be started without delay.
   (b) Since body size is compared to US children of same age, pediatric consultation is not required at this time, and poses a risk in drawing attention to a relatively unimportant child health problem.
   (c) If not already arranged, a pediatric or family practice appointment should be scheduled without delay.
   (d) Lack of documentation of the growth delay suggests that other medical problems also might be omitted in the paperwork provided to the Smiths, and on this basis no further psychiatry or medical evaluation should be attempted until full documentation is received from the host country.
   (e) Since physical growth is a function of emotional nurturance, a "wait and see" approach is appropriate in the new home environment, such that a pediatric appointment could be scheduled in 6–8 months if the growth trajectory does not show improvement.
2. As you are the first psychiatrist to consult on Jorge's care, describe your approach to others on the clinical team.
   (a) Inform Beth and Ted that you will never discuss his treatment with his case manager or therapist unless specifically requested by one of them, in order to preserve Jorge's privacy.
   (b) Explain to the clinical team and the Smiths that your practice is limited to medication management, and that they should only consult you when there is reason to expect that a change in medication treatment will be helpful.
   (c) Offer to provide opinion at any stage of treatment, and suggest availability for ongoing assessment if symptoms change even if there is no clear indication for a new medication.
   (d) Demonstrate leadership by informing the therapist and case manager that you are in charge of the overall care plan, and instruct them that you expect to be notified of any changes in therapy, in the school plan, or in the family.
   (e) Patiently explain to the Smiths that RAD is not a diagnosis which can be treated by psychiatry medications, so instead of consulting psychiatry they should find an expert in RAD who uses novel and specialized techniques that can repair early defects in attachment.

3. Now suppose that in Jorge's first days in kindergarten, the worry about hyperactivity appears to be confirmed by his constant motion, inattention to direction, and refusal to join in quiet group activities. Patient observation confirms that Jorge understands directions but "simply won't follow them. The school has arranged for assignment to a psychotherapist, who describes a good working alliance with Jorge. She politely disagrees with the theory that Jorge has ADHD, she reminds you that any child who has emotional trauma might become overactive in a new setting. Meanwhile, school personnel are urging the Smiths to push harder for treatment of ADHD, and there is some implication that Jorge might not be able to continue in his present kindergarten class "unless something changes." Based on this history, choose your next move in treatment:

(a) ADHD symptom checklists can be administered for two or more settings (such as home and school) to help discern the course of symptoms and for further potential consideration of ADHD.

(b) Since the symptoms presented can be more accurately attributed to the diagnosis of RAD, medications designed to treat ADHD are likely to be unhelpful, and may even paradoxically worsen hyperactivity.

(c) If further psychological testing supports multiple diagnoses such as RAD, ADHD, and PTSD, residential treatment should be considered.

(d) Given the complexity of diagnosis and the uncertain origin of symptoms, a 30-day inpatient diagnostic evaluation is indicated, to include brain imaging and genetic testing.

(e) If Jorge's new therapist is not fluent in Spanish, you should recommend that he be transferred to a new therapist, preferably one who is culturally sensitive and bilingual.

4. You are scheduled to meet again with Jorge, who is now a first grader. The consult question from the school involves the rise in oppositional defiant behavior, such as pushing ahead in line and an incident involving foul language toward a teacher. In session with the Smiths, they reveal a separate disappointment about Jorge's failure to return their affection, and the absence of any gratitude for their efforts to make him part of the family. Their sorrow is now more acute because of the contrast with his over-affection toward his teacher, whom he often greets with hugs and kisses. Jorge's teacher however has confided that she feels increasingly uncomfortable with Jorge's physical affection, and she points out that "it makes the other children laugh at him." Which of the following represents a sound clinical recommendation for the school, supported by attachment theory?

(a) A private conference with the school counselor would be helpful toward understanding what Jorge has learned about the meaning of touch. Once this is accomplished, he should receive further instruction to help him gauge his level of familiarity and overt affection.

(b) To forestall a negative developmental trajectory, a gentle but firm confrontation is indicated, and time out in a corner of the classroom should be applied at the first sign of over-affection.

(c) A neutral adult figure in the school should be assigned to meet and greet Jorge when he arrives at school, in order to provide a warm hug at the start of the day. In addition to satisfying his obvious need for physical affection, this will also provide an experience at the "receiving end" and thereby can help him develop a social sense of touching.

    (d) Whenever Jorge attempts to hug or kiss his teacher, she should turn away, and deliberately show greater interest in other children.

    (e) When Jorge tries to hug or kiss his teacher, adults should carefully abstain from any criticism or expression of concern, so as to reduce the risk of injuring Jorge's fragile, nascent social drive and his beginning effort at attachment.

5. Now consider that Jorge is a second grader and multiple clinical assessments have culminated in diagnosis of RAD. Your mission in this appointment is to address the problem of Jorge's violence in school toward other children, which is sometimes reactive to insult or interference, but in other cases seems to be premeditated. An example is tripping other children on the playground, and teachers have witnessed a careful preparation and some delight in the results of this behavior. Which of the following recommendations to the school would be most likely to enhance the development of *object constancy* for a child with delay of attachment?

    (a) Observation of Jorge in the classroom will lead to an understanding of what he looks like just before starting a fight: at the least sign of violence Jorge should stand in front of the class and apologize for his anger.

    (b) If adults will deliberately ignore Jorge's negative behaviors during his adaptation to school, he will internalize the belief that his acceptance into a group can be unconditional. This sense of security will become the foundation for adhering to a social code as a bona fide member of his peer group.

    (c) In a private session with his principal, this adult should calmly explain that Jorge is not disliked, but that he unfortunately is now at risk for being expelled because of the school's zero tolerance policy for violence.

    (d) In a private session, a counselor or therapist may explain that Jorge can receive help in understanding the feelings that give rise to violence; while at the same time will be accountable for violating rules that apply in class to all the children.

    (e) When correct boundaries are in place, the school's job is to teach and the parents' job is to discipline. The school should encourage Jorge's adoptive parents to punish Jorge however they see fit. School personnel will refrain from any direct correction of bad behavior, but will send home daily reports of violence or rule infractions.

6. Consider that comprehensive evaluation of symptoms in third grade has led to additional diagnosis of ADHD for Jorge, and his behavior improved markedly with trial of a medication treatment for this disorder. While his compliance and cooperation have increased, initial report of academic success is favorable. You are surprised to hear from an inpatient unit, calling to request an appointment to continue outpatient care.

An incident of "wild aggressive behavior" at school and description of mood symptoms has led to provisional diagnosis of childhood-onset bipolar disorder.

There is description of initial improvement in a neuroleptic medication and a recent inpatient trial of an SSRI antidepressant agent. The inpatient therapist who calls you relates the team consensus that Jorge is "getting worse the longer he stays here." There is also concern about an immediate weight gain on the current medications, and some of the staff attribute this to overindulgence and "comfort eating." Describe a best initial response to the request to resume outpatient care.

(a) Since Jorge is gaining weight on a neuroleptic medication, you cannot accept treatment until this medication has a wash-out and a minimum of 2 weeks inpatient observation to verify both stability and maintenance of general health.

(b) Request explanation for start of an antidepressant on the unit and further information about any correlation with the rise in disruptive behavior. Explain that an outpatient appointment can be arranged when Jorge is stable and in control of his behavior.

(c) Firmly decline to accept Jorge as an outpatient while strongly encouraging referral to a residential treatment center in a nearby state, which specializes in treatments of RAD.

(d) Gently probe to see whether the Smiths plan to continue the adoption or would consider a return to foster care with the hope that Jorge could be accepted into a family from his home or a neighboring country.

(e) Inform the inpatient unit that you can accept him into outpatient treatment if you can guide the inpatient medication treatment plan for 1 week prior to his discharge.

7. In your first appointment with Jorge after discharge from inpatient, further perspective is gained from review of the records, a discussion with his therapist, and interview with each family member. Prior to hospitalization, Jorge had revealed to his therapist a partial but very troubling memory of a grown-up who touched him in his "privates," and Jorge feels that this occurred when he was very little but "he remembers it in nightmares." Then during the week after this came out in therapy, Jorge became much more hyperactive and frankly disruptive in class. The same week at home he experimented with building fires in the basement, and the next day his agitation at school culminated in admission to a child inpatient unit. Consider further recommendations based on this more detailed account of the pre-hospital course.

(a) Since the time Jorge confided in his therapist about trauma, his behavior is much worse. On this basis, any further contact with the therapist may itself become traumatic, and hence he should be reassigned to a new therapist after carefully explaining the transition process to him in terms of his understanding.

(b) A specialized treatment center should be consulted which provides for re-birthing and "forced hugs" as potentially required when basic trust has been violated as manifest in the overlapping diagnoses of PTSD with RAD.

(c) Medication treatments specifically designed for post-traumatic symptoms should be considered, and all other medications should be held while monitoring the effect of medication treatment for PTSD symptoms.

(d) Unless detrimental factors of therapy are identified, encourage Jorge and his family to continue with their current therapist but assure them that the therapist will monitor the level of stress and will not force Jorge to reveal or reexperience further troubling memories; check with the therapist about the management of PTSD symptoms in therapy.

(e) Schedule a sleep study for Jorge in order to ensure that problems of sleep architecture are not the actual cause for the nightmares about trauma.

8. You are asked by a pediatrician to provide a consult for another case, a girl Jane who is now age 7 and carries diagnoses of both ADHD and RAD. She was removed from her biological family in another state, "before age 2," and soon after as a toddler Jane received diagnosis of RAD (clinical records not available). She has had four foster home placements. Your colleague in pediatrics reports that Jane is increasingly prone to episodes of rage, which include head banging and "screaming at the top of her lungs." The consult question is to rule out early onset bipolar disorder.

Further history from her case manager and from records reveals that Jane also has social and verbal delays, which are long standing. Since transfer to her current foster home 2 years ago, Jane has yet to develop a friendship with a same-age child. She does not play and turns away from other children when approached. She enjoys a solitary activity she calls knitting, but the behavior actually involves a peculiar stretching out of napkins, and she seems content with this until repeatedly urged to shift her behavior. Rage episodes commonly begin with the request to interrupt "knitting," but have also occurred in reaction to loud noises and to changes in daily routine. Her teacher observes that the anger is hard to predict because Jane speaks in a monotone and shows little facial expression to warn of an incipient "explosion." Overall, the anger episodes "seem to be getting much worse." Describe the best initial approach to diagnosis:

(a) Both RAD, inhibited type, and autistic spectrum disorder (ASD) should be diagnosed based on the information provided.

(b) Since the definition of RAD, inhibited type, covers the current syndrome, no further evaluation is indicated for diagnostic purposes.

(c) If on evaluation all the diagnostic criteria are met for ASD, diagnosis should be changed to ASD in place of RAD.

(d) Since symptoms of the inhibited type of RAD are more persistent than those of the disinhibited type of RAD, continuing quasi-autistic symptoms are to be expected.

(e) The form and rage are evidence of childhood bipolar disorder, which can be added to the diagnostic formulation while retaining the current diagnosis of RAD, inhibited type.

9. A 5-year-old child, Timmy, is brought to you by his parents on advice of his kindergarten teacher because of his hyperactivity in school and his disruption of class when he has to share or take turns. During a separate interview with his parents Timmy plays quietly with a member of the office, but on spying his parents returning to the waiting room he pushes over the castle he has made with blocks, runs out the door, then immediately rushes back to his mother and hugs

her leg so fiercely that she is almost dragged down. When she tries to reassure and at the same time acquire her balance, Timmy responds with a look of angry resentment. Based on this limited frame of reference, which of the following best applies as a preliminary conclusion about Timmy's behavior?

(a) This is a normal or expectable reaction to separation from parents at this age, since this essentially comprises a "strange situation" test of attachment.

(b) Timmy is likely to have an insecure-disorganized type of attachment.

(c) Reactive attachment symptoms are suggested by the ambivalent, indiscriminate and intense display of emotion.

(d) Timmy shows a secure attachment to his mother, and though he was distracted by play in the waiting area, he remembers his fears of separation when his parents came into view.

(e) ADHD symptoms were quiescent until arrival of his parents, at which point an overload of emotional stimuli caused him to lose control.

10. While waiting to see his pediatrician, Tommy, age 3, regards with interest how all the adults are absorbed in looking at magazines. He tries to grab one himself off the table but accidentally knocks over a lamp. His mother quietly sets the lamp back in place and then offers him a magazine, turning to a colorful picture. Which of the following is best represented?

(a) The substituted gesture

(b) Pseudomaturity

(c) The facilitated gesture

(d) Symbiosis

(e) Misattunement

Chapter 3
Theories for the Origin of RAD

Part 1: Biological Basis

Genetic Coding of Attachment

By definition, RAD requires the critical influence of grossly pathogenic care in early childhood. Yet, not all children exposed to neglect develop a generalized social impairment. Attachment behavior may actually increase in the context of emotional deprivation as sadly evident in the child who clings tightly to a parent figure who is known to be neglectful, or abusive. Biological factors can thus be considered either vulnerability to pathogenic care or, in terms of the resilience displayed by those children who seem to have protection against negative influences, even at critical stages of development [68].

We have no pedigrees to elucidate the degree of heritability of factors for vulnerability or resilience for RAD; however, the subtypes of attachment have been studied for direction of genetic influence, following the standard paradigm of the Strange Situation. Finkel and Matheny [69] have demonstrated high concordance for attachment classification for monozygotic (N=99) vs. dizygotic (N=108) twins. Other research have mainly focused on the subtype of disorganized attachment, because of its link to childhood psychopathology. A major breakthrough in genetics is the work by Gervai et al. [70], who report high frequency of the 7-repeat allele of the DRD4 gene in 12-month-olds classified as disorganized in attachment by the Ainsworth Strange Situation test. DNA was harvested from cheek cell samples of 91 family trios (parents and child) and three mother–infant pairs. Parents heterozygous for the 7-repeat allele of DRD4 transmitted this allele nonrandomly to infants classified as disorganized. Conversely, the transmission rate was lower than chance for those infants classified as securely attached. Gervai et al. point out that DRD4 gene codes for dopamine receptors, which increase in density especially at the period of 6–12 months of age.

D.F. Shreeve, *Reactive Attachment Disorder: A Case-Based Approach*,
SpringerBriefs in Child Development, DOI 10.1007/978-1-4614-1647-0_3,
© Springer Science+Business Media, LLC 2012

Discovery of a relationship of the DRD4 gene to attachment is remarkable also because polymorphism of the DRD4 gene is linked to ADHD [71]. Though this is not in itself proof of a common underlying basis, it is probable that both attachment and the faculty of sustaining attention require intact dopamine pathways of the pre-frontal cortex. Clausen et al. [72] hypothesize a common origin in infant development for the faculty of attachment and joint attention, observing that "positive inter-subjectivity with others is a major fulcrum around which early disruption of social skill revolves in infants with coherent attachment strategies." Infants with disorganized attachment, in this view are those with deficient capacity to "establish episodes of positive inter-subjectivity with others", and the related failure of joint attention modifies the subsequent "relationship of attachment to language and cognitive outcomes."

Epigenetic Models

An animal (rodent) model for gene-environment interactive effect on attachment is available in the phenomenon of relationship between maternal nurturing behavior and stress-tolerance of offspring in the postnatal period. Weaver et al. [73] identified high-nurturing mother rats by their high incidence of licking and grooming (LG). Pups of such mothers are known to show small hypothalamo-pituitary (HPA) responses to novel stresses [74]. This endocrine effect of maternal nurturance appears to be mediated by a block on methylation of the promoter region of the gene for glucocorticoid receptors (GR). Since methylation blocks transcription of the GR promoter region, the net effect of the block on methylation by high maternal nurturance increases the number of GR receptors on the hippocampus. This promotes feedback control over the HPA axis, in turn reducing the rise of cortisol with stress. Though nature's mechanism for stress tolerance appears to be intricate, the outcome is effective in rendering greater stress tolerance for pups raised by highly nurturing mothers. A proof for this epigenetic mechanism is the reversal of stress protection by cross-fostering of pups: those born of high LG mothers lose the protective damp-ening of the HPA response, when raised by low LG mothers. In a further demonstration of physiologic mechanism, the authors demonstrate that pharmacologic manipulation of DNA methylation can block the effect of high maternal nurturance on the set point for the HPA axis response to stress.

Bagot and Meaney [75] summarize the field of animal research which now links maternal nurturing (licking and grooming behavior for the female rat) and the set-point of neonatal HPA axis mediated through "environment x gene interaction." High rate of LG, for example, in the neonatal period modifies endocrine as well as cardiovascular response to stress. Experimental manipulation of the pups – such as grooming with a brush in the first week of life – increases hippocampal GR density and dampens the HPA response to stress. Likewise, interventions which increase stress in the mother result in a decrease in LG behavior, and thus lead to a decrease in hippocampal GR density, thereby increasing HPA sensitivity. Pups of mothers with the low LG trait are also prone to behavioral inhibition evidenced, for example, by decreased exploration. They are sensitive to fear conditioning. Compared to other epigenetic effects, maternal down-regulation of HPA sensitivity in the postnatal period is also remarkably enduring and in fact affects parental behavior of the next generation, an effect termed by Bagot and Meaney as "social imprint."

In a striking parallel to research on epigenetic programming in animals, Lakotos et al. [76] report a significant association between attachment disorganization in human infants and polymorphism of the dopamine receptor gene DRD4 (specifically the DRD4 III exon 48 bp repeat polymorphism). Spangler et al. [77] were not able to replicate these findings in subsequent research, but instead discovered an association between infant disorganized attachment (defined by the Strange Situation at 12 months) and the short allele polymorphism of the serotonin transporter gene (s/s form of the 5-HTTLPR polymorphism). This research demonstrates an epigenetic effect similar to the animal model: the predisposed genotype is activated by a condition of maternal low sensitivity, as measured by separate observational scales of maternal response to infant signals. For infants of mothers who fell into the "low responsiveness" group, the homozygous short allele genotype of 5-HTTLPR carried significant risk for disorganized attachment (categorized by the Strange Situation at 12 months). Apart from the criteria of the Strange Situation test used in the study, level of security of attachment did not independently associate with genotype. The authors conclude that the epigenetic effect is mediated by features which correlate with attachment, namely, emotion regulation and attention capacity during stress (the Strange Situation can thus be regarded as a kind of infant stress test). Spangler et al. remark the previous discovery of relationship of the short allele genotype to other measures of stress susceptibility in humans and propose that the vulnerability in infants with the short allele to maternal insensitivity has a probabilistic (rather than determinative) effect on attachment.

Biological Effect of Maternal Stress

Stress-induced hormonal change has long been suspected as a cause for defective maternal attachment behavior in mammals. Mammal physiology provides for a dampening down of the HPA axis in the perinatal period, presumed to be the normal state in humans as well as other mammals [78]. An animal model involves the modulation of neuro-endocrine and behavioral responses to stress both in pups and their mothers, during the critical postnatal period; central mechanisms filter stimuli that are not relevant to primary functions of the perinatal period, (namely, feeding and attachment). Female rats in the late gestation, parturition, and lactation phases show marked reduction in HPA response to a range of stressful stimuli such as noise, immobilization, and the "swim test." Walker et al. [78] propose that in humans as well as other mammals, down-regulation of endocrine stress response in the perinatal period is protective of CNS development for the neonate. The authors speculate that impingement on this physiological down-regulation could play a role in postpartum depression, while also interfering with the process of attachment of mother and newborn.

Talge et al. [79] illustrate an additional mechanism for maternal stress effects on attachment, which is mediated by cortisol. Cortisol crosses the placenta, and in animal models there is correlation of maternal and fetal cortisol (though fetal cortisol changes only as a fraction of the change in maternal cortisol in maternal stress). The authors propose a possible, adaptive role for high maternal cortisol in up-regulating neonatal HPA reactivity and thereby promoting hypervigilance, which could be critically important for those young born under conditions which are sufficiently stressful to mothers to promote high cortisol in the prenatal period. Talge et al. propose that high stress exposure of modern living actually activates the stress reactivity of the newborn and thereby predisposes to anxiety disorder, to language delay, and to Attention Deficit Hyperactivity Disorder. The authors hypothesize that for humans, prenatal up-regulation of stress response may have increased biological fitness in the primordial past, during phases of adverse environmental conditions, whereas in modern times the effects of high maternal cortisol are uniformly deleterious; "they exist today at the cost of vulnerability to neurodevelopmental disorders."

In humans – as well as in other mammals – maternal stress could of course also directly interfere with maternal competence in care giving. Martins and Gaffan [80] provide a meta-analysis of six studies of human maternal depression, which together reveal that infants of mothers who suffer depression early in pregnancy show significantly less likelihood of secure attachment, as measured in their offspring by the Ainsworth Strange Situation. There is parallel increase in both insecure avoidant and disorganized attachment. Other related research have shown postpartum depression to be associated with both delayed cognitive development and insecure attachment, particularly in boys [81, 82]. Shaw and Vondra [83] have found that, presumably as a function of maternal stress, low-income mothers and their infants have high rates of attachment insecurity, with correlative increase in externalizing symptoms by age 3. Maternal depression, difficult temperament, and low maternal involvement each predict behavior problems in late childhood, especially for boys.

Even though maternal stress and depression significantly affect type of attachment, there is comparatively less information about how these antenatal factors could impact upon Reactive Attachment Disorder itself. In theory, the emotional withdrawal implicit in severe postpartum depression could present an influence similar to neglect, but for RAD, "grossly pathogenic care" is necessary. Research on antenatal causes of attachment disorder is confounded by the number of variables that apply to contexts of extreme deprivation, and the cumulative stress factors that impinge upon mothering under conditions of hardship. Young maternal age and high emotional stress, for example, may overlap poverty effects including malnutrition. Low birth weight can independently affect the course of early attachment [23].

Since substance abuse disorder is a known prenatal risk factor, prenatal cocaine exposure has also been considered for its potential effect on attachment. Research demonstrates, however, that level of cocaine exposure does not predict attachment type. Beeghly et al. [84] report that "contrary to popular perceptions, level of prenatal cocaine exposure was not significantly related to secure/insecure attachment status, disorganized attachment status, or rated level of felt security." Viewed from a different perspective, the finding that maternal depression is more predictive of attachment disorder than prenatal cocaine exposure emphasizes the importance of preventive mental health during pregnancy and points toward early intervention in maternal affective illness.

Maturation and Lesions of Early Limbic Pathways

Some of the brain regulatory structures which sustain life are mature at birth: these are primarily those controlling breathing in the medulla, and may be termed truly "hard wired." Joseph [85] observes that centers within the human limbic system which govern emotional regulation are immature at birth and in fact experience expectant, that is, the growth and differentiation of the amygdala, cingulate gyrus, and septal nuclei require the emotionally intense interactions, which characterize the dyad in infancy. Brain growth – specifically the growth and connectivity of the limbic nuclei – is a direct function of attachment experience in the first 3 years, according to Joseph. Joseph's is a "use or lose" model, in that continuous and active interactions, imbued with affect and defining relationship, become a foundation of a capacity to respond interpersonally at subsequent points, throughout the lifespan. Conversely, the Joseph model predicts that emotional neglect at critical periods of infancy and early childhood are catastrophic for brain centers that mediate human socio-emotional response.

By reference to animal research, and using human case examples, Joseph illustrates that severe emotional deprivation in infancy leads to atrophy of critical limbic structures, or to pathological mal-development of limbic networks with autonomic and cortical areas: he compares this to animal experiments which demonstrate degeneration of the visual cortex when one eye is covered at birth. (Brain networks corresponding to the blind eye are replaced by those which respond to visual input in the contralateral eye.) According to this understanding of limbic development, if sufficient stimuli of the right kind are not provided in critical periods of infancy and toddlerhood – as in conditions of severe neglect and pathogenic care – neurons of limbic structures "will establish or maintain aberrant, abnormal connections, or whither, die, and drop out at an accelerated rate." The effect predicted by Joseph is not subtle: he estimates from animal studies that severe neglect could decrease the number of synapses per neuron a thousand fold, and can "retard the growth and eliminate billions, if not trillions of synapses per brain...in summary, early social and environmental influences exert significant organizing effects not only on the brain but shape and mold all aspects of intellectual, perceptual and emotional development."

Presumably to offset such catastrophic effects on brain development, powerful drives serve to protect attachment during the critical window of opportunity for limbic development. To further his thesis on limbic mal-development in humans, Joseph turns to the pioneering ethological studies of rhesus monkeys by Harlow and

Harlow [86]. Joseph illustrates that in the rhesus monkey model, un-mothered young will form indiscriminate emotional attachment to wire frames, inanimate objects, and even other species that are natural predators. Reflecting the intergenerational effect of limbic mal-development, mother rhesus monkeys which were themselves deprived of emotional nurturance at the infant stage show subsequent indifference or even hostility toward their own young and will "brutalize them, biting off fingers and toes, pounding them, and nearly killing them…" (until caretakers intervene; [87]).

Since infant limbic structures mature at different rates, differential effects correspond to the timing of pathogenic care. Animal studies again support this thesis: surgical ablation of limbic structures reveals their characteristic "signature." The amygdala is first to mature, and in humans the process begins in the first year. Bilateral amygdala destruction in animals or bilateral destruction by disease in humans produces emotional blunting and social disinterest. Humans with amygdala lesions, as described by Joseph "cease to respond in appropriate, social, emotional, or motivational characteristics of their environment." In ablation experiments in animals, the amygdala – without other limbic centers – reveals an intense craving for social contact which is nonselective; thus Joseph concludes the undifferentiated social drive is an initial amygdala feature, even though in later childhood myelination of the medulla transforms the amygdala to an organ which coordinates with other limbic structures in promoting selective attachment, and even inhibition of gregarious responses.

Joseph observes that, from the perspective of developmental neurophysiology, the critical period for each limbic center reveals itself in a superabundance of synapses, in preparation for synaptic pruning, according to the Joseph model. Based on this postulate, relatively late-maturing limbic centers begin their differentiation by 8–10 months. Based on animal results, the limbic septal nuclei have a primary role in selective, differential response and inhibit the general social drive. With some resemblance to the disinhibited form of RAD, laboratory animals with ablation of septal nuclei are governed by their contact-loving amygdala, and demonstrate an oral, indiscriminant nature oddly overlapping an aggressive nature, which Joseph depicts as "bullying." In behavioral terms, maturation of septal nuclei and the late myelination of amygdala can be measured in terms of differential response to known vs. unknown persons, in particular in the emergence of "stranger anxiety." Thus by 9 months 70% of children respond negatively to approach of a stranger, and by 1 year, 90% respond aversively, as a combined influence of the mature amygdala (now promoting wariness), the cingulate gyrus, and the gradually maturing septal nuclei.

Joseph also proposes a means by which deprivation stress may damage the critical limbic matrix. High cortisol and enkephalins are neurotoxic in high stress states, whereas high norepinephrine (NE) tone – characteristic of emotional security – is neuro-protective, and growth promoting. Overactivation of the hippocampus and limbic structures, according to Joseph, depletes NE and thereby interferes not only with emotional interactions but with development of memory, which is so essential to remembering history of particular social relationships, and applying socio-emotional context to new experience.

Schore [88] builds upon the Joseph model of limbic development, but expands its application to a synthesis of the fields of attachment and emotion regulation in infancy. In a remarkable synthesis, Schore incorporates Bowlby's attachment, Mahler's stages of separation-individuation and modern understandings of emotion regulation into a study of the physiology and anatomy of the developing human brain. A starting point to approach Schore's work on the subjects of emotional regulation and attachment is to consider the role of the right brain: it is the right hemisphere according to theory which is dominant for attachment, and it is attachment behavior which organizes control over emotion regulation [89]. Attachment and emotional regulation devolve together, in the setting of dyadic experience. The infant's right hemisphere according to this model is synchronized through interactive behavior with the mature right cortical hemisphere of its mother, who interprets, reflects, and shares the infant's discovery of the world. In the healthy dyad, a dynamic, synchronous, and joyful attunement prevails in the first year, according to Schore, and this hedonic state is growth facilitating, favoring neuro-proliferation and especially a differentiation of the right prefrontal cortex which maintains and organizes a neural network for attachment, linked to autonomic, limbic, and other cortical areas.

The process of attachment begins (according to the Schore model) with the child's motivation to enter into a reciprocal reward system characterized by a "self-maintaining vitality externally regulated by the psychobiologically attuned mother." The corresponding, major task for the first year is therefore development of a tolerance for affective arousal that characterizes the hedonic state of merger. The merger is a "crucible for the forging of preverbal affective ties." Key maternal functions during the second and third quarter of the first year – which Schore compares to Mahler's phase of symbiosis – involve co-experiencing and mirroring back of the child's positive affect, as well as tempering and modulating of negative affects. High dopamine levels favor transcription of genes which encode precursors of endorphins, and high endogenous opiates predispose to heightened sympathetic tone which mediates a predominantly positive affect, favoring a state of alertness and activation. High sympathetic tone also promotes neuroproliferation and brain organization, especially that of the prefrontal cortex, which Schore presents as the chief organizing center for attachment.

Under the mother's watchful gaze, the first experiments with crawling or ambulating way engender a kind of self-celebration and embrace of life opportunity, identified as the Practicing Phase of separation-individuation in Mahler's model of separation-individuation. This period of 9–16 months is hedonic (pleasurable) as depicted by Schore, and mediated by dopaminergic tone as well as endorphin influence. The predominant affect is certainly reinforced by maternal mirroring of her child's joy, displayed in prosody of speech and with glad facial expressions in the fun moment of exploration. Trips back to the mother for "refueling" may involve, according to Schore, a kind of real-time "micro-regulation," literally a split-second visual contact which operates to synchronize right hemisphere states of arousal for mother and infant, the physiologic equivalent of emotional re-attunement.

A potential, important challenge to attunement emerges in the late Practicing Phase, when at around 18 months the infant's advancing capacity to move away from close supervision raises the likelihood of a mishap, or simply getting lost. At an emotional level, advancing mobility demonstrates awareness of physical separateness from the mother and hence, the dawning of separation anxiety. Schore surmises that in this phase a uniformly applauding response of the mother's celebration of movement shifts rather abruptly to a pattern of frequent prohibitions and sanctions, necessary to the prevention of accidents, and also intrinsic to the first enforcement of rules such as apply to what may be put in the mouth or how toileting is to be managed. The infant experiences the shock of negative maternal appraisal, a potentially catastrophic and disorganizing event, in effect a sudden loss of attunement, which results in the discovery of shame. As explained by Schore, however, the discovery of this new emotion is also the root of socialization for emotional response. In fact it is repair of attunement through maternal reframing and supervision which provides the infant with a model for emotional regulation. To summarize, the mother's rejection of the infant's direction of action and interest causes a rejection experience, which however can then immediately be repaired by management of the induced, negative affect by redirection and through comforting. The net effect is to renew the dyadic attachment, thus establishing a rhythm of re-attunement.

Identification with the mother's capacity to regulate negative affect and a growing faith in reliable rescue become foundations for emotional self-regulation. A repeated, comanaged repair of misattunement also inspires a belief in the availability of the mother at crucial moments, which becomes an internal working model for management of negative affect that applies to independent experience. That is, the belief that help can apply to trouble derives from dyadic experience but is useful later in promoting a separate organized response to negative emotional experience. At the physiological level Schore proposes that the schema for management of negative affect depends upon maturation of the prefrontal cortex, and its link to the right cortical representational system.

In the ensuing separation phase of rapprochement, and progressing to object constancy, images of self and other can apply in times of crisis, and the memory of partnership in resolving distress. A capacity for independent management of emotions progresses with unconscious retrieval of memories that provide for experiences of interaction with others and in the implicit memory of effective coping with new situations of distress. The accretion of implicit "relational" memories therefore applies directly to the child's growing capacity to regulate emotion. Attachment beyond the dyad builds upon strength of the dyad and stability of the sense of self, such that security and the associated implicit memories of dyadic partnership apply to increasingly higher levels of social relationship.

In the moment of shame, according to the Schore model, a parasympathetic tone prevails, interrupting the sympathetically mediated hedony of the Practicing Phase of separation-individuation. Failure to rescue on the part of the parent (usually the mother) is held to be at the core of psychopathology in early childhood. When the mother lacks ability to re-attune after applying limits to joy, interactive repair of shame is not possible. Empathic failure, or the mother's repeated, inadequate handling of moments of distress carries a high cost as "extensive dysregulating experiences...permanently etched into forming cortical-subcortical circuits in the form of right-hemispheric pathological representations of self-in-interaction-with-a-dysregulating other." Shame persists as an internalization, and the failure in attachment is matched equally by disability in regulation of emotion. Physiologically, Schore postulates that the model predicts abnormal persistence of parasympathetic tone in the condition of insecure avoidant attachment, such that new (and potentially corrective) interpersonal experience is less available.

Another proposition of Schore is that normal development of emotions regulation depends further upon the elaboration of an interconnecting right cortical, limbic, and autonomic (somatic) emotions systems which together function to "mediate the adaptive capacity of empathetically perceiving the emotional states of other humans beings." New experience in the normal state of secure attachment involves a moment of sympathetic arousal, followed by rise of parasympathetic tone, a sequence which can represent the process of coping and accommodation "as soon as the context is appraised as safe." This capacity is regulated by higher limbic structures and the orbitofrontal cortex (primarily right hemispheric). Normal resolution of stress response thus depends upon implicit memory of safety in attachment, a right-lateralized cortical function of the developing brain.

Stress Tolerance and the Developing Brain

Schore has also proposed a model for trauma effect on developing integration of cortical, limbic, and autonomic networks [89]. In the traumatized child, the implicit memory of "safe through secure attachment" may not be available and cannot be accessed for the autonomic process of recovery from over-arousal. The traumatized, dysregulated child may be progressively prone to "forfeit potential opportunities for socio-emotional learning during critical periods of right brain development." Schore depicts the traumatized child as overwhelmed by surges of intense emotion that then interfere with organization of responses, such that loss of homeostasis interferes with executive function.

Teicher et al. [90] present a parallel theory for the effect of trauma on early brain development which proposes that early maltreatment and stress may produce a physiological "cascade of events" culminating in impairment in CNS development in traumatized children. The authors propose that stress-induced elevations of cortisol and vasopressin-oxytocin impair neurogenesis, myelination, and the elaboration of synapses during sensitive periods of development. An ultimate cost for the exposed young brain is reduced size or function of the corpus callosum, left neocortex, hippocampus, and amygdala, according to the authors. Stress effects on limbic structures and their pathways to neocortex (and possibly cerebellar vermis) may predispose to childhood PTSD, ADHD, and borderline personality to dissociative states while also impinging upon the capacity for normal social responses.

Van der Kolk and Saporta [91] propose a related model for trauma effects on the developing limbic system, which involves a theory of limbic overload, which impacts upon the developmental path of the temporal cortex, culminating in effects on personality. The authors remark that limbic structures which process the emotional cues and which assign valence of incoming signals normally form links with the locus coeruleus, the anatomical core of physiological arousal. Persistent high arousal predisposes to defensive responses, despite a general numbing of reaction to new experience. Memory capacity itself is damaged by the trauma experience as "severe or prolonged stress can disrupt hippocampal functioning, creating context-free fearful associations which are hard to locate in space and time." The authors also predict that intermittent stimulation of the limbic system (by over-arousal and trauma) may alter neuronal thresholds, with effects on development of the temporal lobe that cause personality dysfunction.

Joseph's model of permanent damage to limbic structures is an important starting point in the science of attachment physiology, but the actual improvement of many children now raises doubt about whether there is so direct a comparison to limbic ablation experiments in animals. The evidence favors a view of trauma in early childhood as fundamentally different from adult PTSD. For a child's plastic and relatively flexible limbic cortex, sustained and repetitive emotional trauma impacts on the growth and interconnectedness of brain centers. The abilities to formulate and verbally process are less developed in childhood, and these abilities become actual casualties of the traumatic experience. Trauma in childhood presumably also impairs the capacity to manage further trauma; residual symptoms may be determined by the viability of attachment.

Physiological Measurement of Attachment Disorder

Investigations of physiological events which correspond to attachment behavior are few, but these few show promise, especially in the study of stress tolerance, and in study of autonomic physiology. An example is measurement of the rise in parasympathetic tone which occurs with reunion after separation in healthy children. Respiratory sinus arrhythmia (RSA) is a relatively pure marker of parasympathetic tone (as compared, e.g., to heart rate, which has reciprocal sympathetic and parasympathetic control). With the stress of separation and reunion in the Strange Situation, Oosterman and Shuengel [92] found that foster children with high scores on the Disturbances of Attachment Interview showed relatively high scores for RSA on reunion with unfamiliar caregivers, but an overall low autonomic variation in the Strange Situation.

A perspective on attachment physiology is also provided by comparison of physiological measures of stress to behaviors linked to attachment. As an example, for secure children introduced to day-care, the extent of crying and protest correlates with cortisol level, whereas for insecure children cortisol is relatively uncoupled from protest behavior (crying) and also is persistently elevated during the early phase of separation. Thus the physiological measure of stress is at least in part uncoupled from visible evidence of distress [93]. Similarly, secure infants show consistency of heart rate elevation and distress (such as crying), with separations on the Strange Situation, whereas insecure-resistant infants show discrepancy between distress behavior and heart rate response, but extend the behavioral signs of protest after physiological recovery. Insecure-avoidant infants often show minimal behavioral distress in the Strange Situation despite significant increase in heart rate and cortisol level [94].

Part 2: Psychological Factors

A Deficit Model

The classic research by Rene' Spitz [95] in European orphanages brought to the world an awareness of the devastating effect of emotional neglect. Children of the Foundling Home were isolated in glass cubicles open at one end, and received doctor or nursing visits 2–3 times per day but had very little other personal contact. The infants remained in their cubicles as long as 18 months (in the comparison site, they moved to shared bedrooms). In this context of extreme interference with attachment, Spitz discovered a unique infantile form of depression, superficially resembling adult depression in its stage of "weepy withdrawing behavior…replaced by a sort of frozen rigidity." The process culminated in utter dejection as "now these children would lie or sit with wide-open expressionless eyes, frozen immobile face, and a faraway look, as if in a daze… contact with children who had reached this stage became increasingly difficulty, and finally impossible."

Borrowing from Sigmund Freud's term "anaclitic" (leaning on) attachment, Spitz defined "anaclitic depression" as the infantile state, superficially resembling the listless appearance of adult depression but specifically related to loss of contact with the mother at a time she is first comprehended as a separate, real person, who can come and go and is distinguishable from a "target" for the gratification of oral need. Spitz defined "pre-object" relations as the dawning awareness of self, inherently related to subjective needs and "other" (the parent figure) as the satisfying need. Progress in differentiation of self and other necessarily depends upon a model for relationship Spitz argued, in turn founded on reliable responses of the parent. These responses are interpreted first in terms of need fulfillment, and gradually as defining the pattern of emotional relationship. Deprived of this differentiation of self and other – which we would now call object constancy – Spitz hypothesized that the infant or child would cease to "cathect" (to invest emotionally) in any new person, or even to show interest in the environment. Spitz proposed that anaclitic depression resembles adult depression only in superficial appearance, since its etiology is specifically determined by loss of the primary love object in very early life, and in its natural course it proceeds to a state of detachment, apathy, and morbid physical decline.

In comparison to what is known about etiology of RAD it is critical to remember that Spitz believed that anaclitic depression required a previous attachment to a mother figure, in addition to the experience of loss. He applied the term "hospitalism" more globally to describe the arrest in development seen in some orphanages at the time: for the most extreme conditions he proposed that "the evil effect of institutional care on infants" led to general arrest of development (which included stunting of intellectual growth) and to "very high mortality [96]." Spitz remarked that "in affected young children, one of the most striking factors was the change in the pattern of reaction to strangers in the last third of the first year...[it] could vary from extreme friendliness to any human partner...to a generalized anxiety expressed in blood curdling screams."

In a recent review of anaclitic depression, Guedeney [97] proposes that the condition characterized by Spitz should more appropriately be classified as a subtype of attachment disorder (rather than as an affective disorder). He suggests (translating from French) that "depression of infancy appears.., to be akin to a protective reaction of the child formed in the context of a specific pathogenic context, as a type of learned helplessness." As explained by Guedeny, the earliest relationship, if it ends in loss, becomes the precedent for the unconscious anticipation of a poor return on investment in relationship. Morbid symptoms identified by Spitz (insomnia, anorexia, and immobility) are interpreted by Guedeny as elements of a combined psychological and physical process; "the traditional distinction between organic growth retardation and nonphysical effects on growth may be mistaken."

In more recent times, children like those treated by Spitz have been evaluated in the large-scale longitudinal study of the English and Romanian Adoptees (ERA) Team [98]. During the Ceausescu regime in Romania, children assigned to orphanage care endured similar harsh conditions and extreme emotional deprivation at critical stages of development. Projects of the ERA Study Team follow the longitudinal course of the neglected children following adoption into good homes in the UK, with UK adoptees serving as a control. The Romanian children adopted into UK families showed persistent signs of a disinhibited attachment disorder, as defined by criteria such as "wandering off," "too friendly with strangers," and "lack of understanding social boundaries." [98] When duration of orphanage care was greater than 6 months, symptoms persisted to the time of surveys at 6 and 11 years, supporting a hypothesis of exposure effect at critical developmental period. There is correlation of attention deficit disorder with disinhibited attachment, and early institutional rearing predicted ADHD as a late childhood diagnosis [99]. Also found are trends to lower IQ as well as prominence of childhood conduct problems, in comparison to children not exposed to pathogenic care. Results suggest a phenomenon of "neurodevelopmental programming during critical periods of development."

The Application of Joint Attention to Attachment

Perhaps the human motive to communicate is founded upon an even more basic drive to establish intersubjective awareness that is so evidently essential to attachment, and hence becomes a biological necessity. The process of sharing affective cues, beginning with the infant's dyadic experience, subsequently expands into a broader social field, in which social cognition is increasingly tested and improved. Tronick and Weinberg [100] hypothesize that even the child's drive to explore the physical world is contingent upon a foundation of intersubjectivity, since discovery depends upon a "mutual construction of meaning." The infant infers meaning of their discoveries of the physical world from the parental observation and response to their explorations. The foundation for the child's appraisal of objects, and of their action upon objects, is a "dyadic consciousness": involving both shared meanings and "mutual regulatory experience" [100]. Systematic research on the exchange of nonverbal signals between infant and parent reveal a surprising elaboration of the human communicative capacity prior to employment of symbolic language. In turn this suggests that the roots of psychopathology may, at least in part, be traced back to the earliest distortions of primitive and preverbal understanding [101–104]. Trevathen [104, 105] illustrates how early social experience may impact upon growth of the brain, such that the preverbal communicative experiences of early infancy directs and regulates the pattern of brain differentiation toward a normal (or abnormal) capacity for reciprocal social response.

It is easy to imagine how the sharing of a positive experience is rewarding for the child, because of the parent's evident enjoyment in "co-discovery." For example, a child points to a toy, the parent smiles appreciatively, and communicates by their tone of voice that they are observing, enjoying, and perhaps willing to engage in the child's play with something new. But equally, a capacity to enter into intersubjective states is the early foundation for the child's regulation of negative emotions when exploration is disappointing, or involves adverse consequence. The child attends to the parent when thwarted, and depending on the adult for reassurance, is able to dampen negative emotional experience. Thus the enjoyment of rewarding experience with the surround – and remedy to negative affect – depends upon the infants growing capacity for joint attention. Joint attention develops from the capacity for intersubjectivity. Moreover, the contingent responses of parent and infant form memories and become internalized as a history of dyadic relationship.

Sharing of mutual experience, though potentially voluntary, must generally escape conscious awareness in early life, as the skill in this capacity is well established within the stage in which implicit memory prevails over verbal representation. We may define joint attention operationally, however, and it may be considered as the ability to share in a focus of interest, as viewing an object or sharing in a discrete activity in a shared moment. In context of the dyad – a model for future relationship – the involvement in a shared subject of interest is the product of a coinciding motivation to focus on a subset of the environmental stimuli that are potentially available.

Objective, quantitative studies of infant capacity for joint attention demonstrate a relationship to attachment. Morales et al. [106] demonstrate that the gaze-following skill of infants at 6 months predicts subsequent "higher level collaborative attention" at 24 months, as measured by the duration of time sustained in a joint activity with the parent. Surprisingly, gaze-following skill at 6 months also predicts emotion regulation (ER) skills at 24 months, as measured by tests of frustration and forced delay (such as presenting an attractive object and then placing it out of reach). For the study, one measure of ER for 2-year-olds is gesturing to invite a parent into a play activity; other examples include self-soothing (such as mouthing of the hands), diversion (such as shifting gaze to a new field, away from the frustrating context), and comfort-seeking (such as touching the parent or drawing close).

Clausen et al. [72] have proposed that joint attention is a direct product of the care-giving environment; "individual differences in infant joint attention skill reflect, in part, the degree to which joint attention bids have become socially reward-ing for the child." To test this hypothesis the authors studied an at-risk group – 56 infants with prenatal cocaine exposure. Infants at 15 months were classified by type of attachment using the Ainsworth Strange Situation. A video-based test quantified joint attention of the infants, at 12 months and at 18 months. An initial finding was that infants of insecurely attached dyads were less likely than secure parent–child dyads to display either coordinated face-to-face attention or to coordinate attention to objects. A clearer view of the relationship comes from the authors' subdivision of types of joint attention skills into the following subtypes: (1) responding to joint attention, such as capacity to follow direction of gaze; (2) initiating a joint attention skill, a capacity to initiate attention coordination such as showing an object or point-ing; and (3) initiating behavior regulation request, such as by a gesture which elicits aid from the adult in obtaining an object or causing an event.

Quantification of these measures of joint attention revealed that infants generally showed the most improvement over time in the domain of initiating behavior regu-lation. For infants classified with disorganized attachment by the Strange Situation at 6 months, a deficit in joint attention was most pronounced in the domain of initi-ating coordinated attention with others (as measured by actions such as showing, pointing, or making eye contact while manipulating a toy). In sum, for the at-risk infants in the study, those with disorganized attachment scored lowest at subsequent stages of development in the initiation of joint attention.

Clausen et al. conclude that the development of joint attention reflects represen-tational capacities of the infant (capacity to use symbols in communication). Secure development may favor this cognitive advance in the service of social relatedness. Conversely, the authors suggest that impoverishment of joint attention in infancy is a contributing cause (at least in the population of "at-risk" infants) for disorganized attachment.

Avoidance and Detachment

Whereas some children with RAD meet requirements for diagnosis of ADHD, oth-ers specifically neglect interaction with their caregiver, in essence deploying a selec-tive inattention or actual avoidance of engagement. Since natural selection should favor attachment as a survival mechanism, we may reasonably ask "how can avoid-ance of a caregiver be explained as adaptive?" Main and Weston [107] began to explore the function of avoidance, when their further observations using the Ainsworth Strange Situation revealed that even securely attached children often turn away from their parent at the reunion phase, or briefly avoid eye contact. Many of the children engage for a short while in perfunctory, half-hearted play, before acknowledging the presence of their parent and joyfully returning to them. To explore the meaning of the child's pause before reengagement, the authors turn first to an ethological model for avoidance. Here the comparable behavior in many animal species is the "cutoff," discovered and defined by Chance [108] as a means for two members of the same species to remain in close proximity despite a strong instinct to flee, or with arousal of aggressive instincts which would prevent proximity. In a "cutoff" display, for example, in bird species, one individual quickly turns away from its neighbor and adopts a posture opposite to threat display, thereby diminishing both attack or flee impulses simultaneously in the sender and in the receiver of the signal. Tinbergen and Moynihan [109] also describe "cutoff" displays in nature, for example, in black-headed gulls a direct frontal gaze represents territorial threat (accentuated by head markings) whereas an emphatic facing away movement signals "no threat" (and is actually a ritualized element of courtship).

Cutoffs in many species have become ritualized (elaborated over evolutionary time for signal function), and are useful in partnered activities, such as nest-building or caring for the young [108]. Chance also describes "displacement activities" as resolving the same conflict of a drive to approach and to withdraw by diversion of energy into a third, apparently unrelated behavior. This often serves the purpose of maintaining proximity in higher animals: for example, self-preening and grooming behaviors serve to allow two individuals maintain proximity, as these displacement activities have become ritualized to signal "peaceful intention." When we compare this ethological model to humans, and in particular to toddlers at the reunion phase of the Strange Situation, it is easy to see a displacement activity as represented by the child who turns away from their mother upon her return, and appears busily preoccupied by an apparently aimless activity, for a brief moment before turning to the parent and renewing engagement.

Main and Weston [107] analyzed avoidant behaviors in secure vs. insecure toddlers, and compared avoidance to cutoff behaviors, which regulate proximity in animals. They also compared secure to insecure toddlers in degree of avoidance and included observations of children with evidence of maltreatment by their parent figure. Both in insecure dyads and in toddlers subject to derogatory remarks of their parent figure, avoidance upon reunion is abnormally prolonged on the Strange Situation Test. In addition, behavior at reunion is disorganized, characterized, for example, by rushing toward the parent, and then away from them or "around them."

In interpreting avoidance at reunion, Main and Weston appear to find the ethological model to be useful, but incomplete, incomplete because, in terms of Bowlby's tenet that, distress is relieved by proximity. This would predict that a parent's hostility or signs of rejection should actually elicit proximity seeking, to resolve distress. A cycle of escalating approach and withdrawal can be expected if signals of rejection trigger fear in the child. In fact this is the very pattern of disorganized attachment:

the child strives frantically to avoid, and at the same time to draw closer. Main and Weston propose that an "escape" from competing drives to approach and withdrawal is available through emotional detachment. That is, by reducing focus on the parent, and on the emotions of reunion, the child directs attention "elsewhere."

Brief avoidance may normally serve attachment by delaying full reunion until the child has mastered control of separation anxiety and negative affect. In insecure infants, or for children reacting to negative appraisal by their parent, the avoidant behavior is carried to an extreme. Main and Weston point out that "a shift in attention away from a primary attachment figure then means a blotting out or negation of the image of the parent…in a more complete account we might better conceive of thought and behavior as becoming actively re-organized away from the parent and the memory of the parent."

The Phenomenon of Shame

Bowlby coined the expression "bitter protest" to apply to the infant response to even brief separation from a parent figure. To interpret the full meaning of the infant's bitter protest, it is necessary to consider the infant's capacity to recollect an image of the parent or to use recollections of the parent returning as a protection from anxiety. For that matter the infantile sense of time, hence the capacity to postpone reaction to separation is primitive in early life, such that finding comfort in this anticipated reunion, is primitive. We might even expect that, for the young infant a parent figure who has moved out of visual range has effectively "disappeared," except that this effect is mitigated in secure attachment by a procedural memory, the implicit promise of a remedy for distress. The child's own avoidance at reunion could be visualized as "turning the tables" on a parent who has (from an infant perspective) momentarily abandoned, and now must demonstrate a positive intention.

Lewis [110] proposes that the brief gaze aversion of infants, upon reunion with their mother after separation, contains a "mixture of pleasure and some hint of shame." In comparison, the exaggerated avoidance and period of disorganization upon reunion seen in infants and toddlers with insecure attachment is viewed by Lewis to represent "humiliated fury," the archetype of a human reaction at any age to rejection by a loved one. Lewis explains further that "shame is the empathetic experience of the other's rejection of the self." Thus, even for adults who feel a loss of love, risk of shame is a price for attachment. Curiously it involves both anger at the loved one and a longing for closeness. This wish for restitution of course strongly resembles the conflicted behavior portrayed so clearly, and without dissembling, by insecure infants at the reunion phase of the Strange Situation.

In a psychodynamic formulation, Lewis also proposes that "shame….is a temporary ablation of the self" as it serves to maintain the attachment in the particular form of a "vicarious experience of the other's scorn or contempt." A potential application to RAD is Lewis' further assertion that repression of "rageful longings," in the context of shame and rejection, functions as a kind of "anti-attentional" mechanism, by isolating the individual from awareness of either resentment or of the painful longing for the loved one. In terms of its potential application to attachment disorder, a chronic, persistent sense of shame resulting from repeated rejections could become a character trait, and may comprise in a general defense against new relationship.

The Impact of Trauma

Diagnostic precision is important in weighing the contribution of trauma and neglect on manifest symptoms; yet, realistically the same children who are emotionally neglected are often physically or sexually abused. Thus the syndromes PTSD and RAD often overlap clinically. An alternative conceptualization involves both as elements of the syndrome Developmental Trauma Disorder [91], a diagnosis proposed for the condition of children who are victim to multiple incidences of trauma and emotional abandonment at key points of early development. Recurrent trauma at critical periods is presumed to endanger the systems for integrating and recovering from trauma, as the direct effect of trauma itself.

The term "complex trauma" is also invoked to describe a cumulative effect of multiple incidences of direct trauma, as well as indirect trauma such as witness to violence, and lack of emotional support in the aftermath of trauma episodes [111]. Cook et al. [112] depict the potentially devastating effect of complex trauma in childhood: these effects include impulse problems, cognitive and language delays, and even problems of physical coordination. Children are prone to dissociate under pressure of anxiety, and to somaticize anxiety rather than to use words as tools. Difficulty labeling emotions is also listed as a general consequence of complex trauma, aggravating the effects of impulse disorder on social problem-solving. Often the child seems to lack a sense of self, or to harbor a deep self-loathing. Such children strive, according to the authors, to disprove or reverse this negative self-image by exhibiting an indifference to the consequences of social dysfunction. Treatment of complex trauma in childhood necessarily involves each of the symptom domains and according to Cook et al. includes the repair and restoration of "effective working models of attachment."

Part 3: Social Origins

Attachment and Social Impairment

Green [113] proposes a reformulation of RAD based on its similarity to pervasive developmental disorder, particularly in the domain of social cognition. According to the author, attachment disorder arises as an effect of maltreatment on social cognition, in particular as mistaken assumptions about relationship predicated by past experience. RAD is thus conceived as caused by distortion of thoughts, rather than primarily comprised of misattunement of dyadic relationship. This view of RAD as cognitively based supports the author's clinical method of treating both RAD and Pervasive Developmental Disorder (PDD) in a "social development clinic," with emphasis on exploring and reconstructing social understanding in affected children. According to Green, PDD and RAD are both disorders of social cognition, and might be recategorized as subtypes of social-cognitive processing disorder and "might then usefully be considered to lie on a continuum of such disorders within the taxonomy, for instance, with the PDD spectrum."

Important clinical features however divide the two major childhood syndromes. Allowing that a small group of withdrawn RAD children show persistence of quasi-autistic symptoms [22], there is an essential separation of RAD from ASD in the course of social development. Idiosyncratic language and stereotypic movements are generally absent in RAD, most children with RAD can express a full range of emotions by facial expression, voice tone, and nonverbal gesture. These language elements are generally employed in correct context, allowing the moment for a response by the other person in conversation, and thereby promoting the sharing of a common conversational theme. Moreover children with RAD usually demonstrate social referencing, such as by pointing to an object of mutual interest, and they can sustain a topic of shared interest.

Theory of Mind and the False Belief Test

Theory of mind has been described as imputing belief to others, conceptualizing the perspective of others or "mindfulness" of the minds of others. This capacity to appreciate separate points of vantage – including one's own as subjective – could be considered in the section on psychological factors, but it is clearly also a social principal. Deficit in theory of mind has come to define a core social deficit of ASD [114], but it is not to be conceived to be an all-or-none phenomenon; for example, theory of mind improves gradually over the course of early childhood. This human faculty now comprises an active research area, related to attachment research in part because our theory of attachment predicts that early socio-emotional deprivation is an impasse to development of social cognition, one which affects capacity for relationship, even the development of empathy.

Arranz et al. [115] propose an emotional scaffolding for theory of mind in children and the authors adopt a family systems approach to the study of how children identify emotional states in others, and how they come to comprehend a perspective different from their own. In support of interactive relationship as the foundation for theory of mind, their study shows significant superiority in theory of mind scores for children classified as securely attached. A series of tests for this ability is applied to check the conclusions: these range from teacher's reports of social, cognitive, and general development to a formal test, the "False Belief Test," graded at increasing levels of difficulty.

Tarullo et al. [116] have applied the false belief to post-institutionalized, internationally adopted children in their effort to understand deficits (or delays) in social cognition which might be attributable to emotional deprivation. The procedure can be summarized as follows: the interviewer portrays a situation to a child in which a doll sees an object placed in a specific location, and then, without the doll "knowing it," the child sees another doll place the object in a new location. The child must remember where the object was originally placed, recall its new location, and correctly recognize that the first doll has a false belief about the object's location. In this way the child identifies perspective of another, its distinction from reality, and from their own perspective. As explained by the authors, "false belief understanding refers to an appreciation that other people's beliefs may differ both from reality and from one's own perspective."

The study by Tarullo et al. compares post-institutional adopted children to children raised in foster care, and to controls. The post-institutional group fared poorly on the false belief test, of which 42.5% performed below chance, despite their overall success on recognizing emotional faces and their relative success in a test of emotion understanding. The significance of impairment on this test for theory of mind held up when several variables were filtered out, including prenatal exposure to alcohol, prenatal malnourishment, country of origin, age of adoption, and physical abuse. Despite the known relationship between verbal ability and theory of mind, the post-institutionalized group also showed significant deficit in the false belief test, after controlling for verbal ability. The authors note that "even children who have been removed from the adverse rearing environment and acquired a stable responsive caregiver and an enriched home environment may still show a delayed development of false belief understanding." Yet the conclusion from the study is that early emotional deprivation causes delay, rather than deficit. This process occurs as "early social deprivation may interfere with developmental precursors of social cognition, so that the requisite groundwork is not laid for subsequent social cognitive development."

Anticipatory Interactive Planning

Even though objective measures of perspective-taking show impairment in post-institutional children, such children show a fundamental difference from ASD in longitudinal course. There is often a sharp improvement in use of language (nonverbal and verbal) to coordinate social interactions. Ability to comprehend and to communicate state of mind improves in the socially enriched setting, compared to less tractable social deficit of autism. In fact many children with the disinhibited type of RAD may appear socially smooth in conversation, employing a range of facial expressions skillfully, and exhibiting normal expressive gestures and prosody of speech. This progression – often outstripping changes in attachment disorder – presents the challenging question: how can language art develop quickly without the corresponding advance in selective attachment, for which purpose language was "invented"?

A theory of social intelligence, Anticipatory Interactive Planning (AIP), may further illuminate the distinction between RAD and ASD in that though related to theory of mind it entails a longitudinal process of interaction more akin to the phenomenon of attachment. The study of AIP [117] arises from a growing recognition that in higher primates, the tasks inherent in social living are more challenging than those of tool using, and hence have more telling influence on the evolution of our species [118]. For purpose of illustrating AIP, Goody [117] observes that social living requires "anticipation of the actions of others, calculation of short and long term gains, and close attention to signals about the consequences of one's own behavior."

At first glance, AIP seems identical to theory of mind; yet it requires a temporal unfolding, an ongoing mutual responsiveness which elapses over time. AIP, like attachment itself, is intrinsically *transactional*. A ready example is language itself, or rather the process of shared conversation, during which each speaker forecasts the next turn of conversation, and builds a response in anticipation. Conversation might be defined as "joint anticipatory planning," to highlight the fact that AIP is more precisely the cognitive modeling of another's contingent response (necessarily invoking a model also of one's own next response) for the purpose of sustaining a shared direction toward a common goal. A uniquely human aspect of AIP is that simply sharing a theme is often rewarding, in the context of attachment, such that an explicit goal becomes secondary to the purpose of maintaining the continuity of reciprocal responses.

AIP applies at a different level to meet the adaptive requirements of complex society and, humans as well as other higher primates and social animals achieve ability to cognitively model their own and another's interdependence both in real time and in context of the history of relationship. Language is the supreme example of this representation of attachment. Hutchins and Hazlehurst [118] propose that – to the extent that language can be studied as the property of a community, rather than that of an individual; "...shared symbols or form-meaning mappings...cannot be explained by reference to the processes operating in individual minds alone." The human capacity of language of course vastly increases the reach through time of attachment, and its impact on cooperative interaction; indeed it can be asserted that it is the acquisition of a vocal apparatus that can pronounce words – and not the opposable thumb – which has directed the course of human evolution. Language facilitates sustained joint attention, and provides for an explicit definition of intent and purpose. The refined rules of grammar multiply the capacity to make intentions explicit, and serve to place an episode of interaction in time (in actual terms or as a proposed happening). Language sustains collaboration of two individuals when they are physically separate, when the "promise" of shared purpose often still holds. This facet of attachment is so integral to AIP that the general advance in language for most children with RAD presents a kind of paradox: how can language continue to develop independent of progress in attachment? Vygotsky's definition of thought as "internalized language" [119] would suggest congruent lines of social and linguistic development. Social cognition theoretically originates in the evocation of the memory of a guide or mentor which can apply in a context of adversity or challenge (the basis for "self-talk" as a mental aid according to Vygotsky's scaffolding theory). Language would thus seem inseparable from attachment.

Yet, the protean forms of AIP provide examples of how language and attachment may separate in the course of development. AIP, for example, can be used to deceive, a useful device for the very reason that communication relies upon a faith in shared meanings. To maximize comprehension, the assumption is made that others are speaking truthfully. This assumption is also necessary to model our own response to meaning conveyed by another speaker. This is, however, the very reason why lying has such potential power: truth is normally assumed in order to expedite communication. Language may therefore be used to exchange information, or may be exploited for the purpose of deception. Potentially, language is an instrument for control. Distortion of AIP for the purpose of deception has in fact been theorized to be the very root of primate social intelligence, following the theory of "Machiavellian intelligence" [120].

Besides the alternatives of cooperation and deception, a third use of AIP may be still more applicable to RAD: that of evasion. The dialogue between two or more individuals depends upon a context of shared culture and what has gone on before between them. There is a relationship history which is assumed, and assumptions greatly simplify what must be made explicit in order to acquire meaning. At the same time, the past history of shared meanings expands each new shared moment, to make it a part of the pattern of intersubjective experience. Yet these assumptions of shared meaning are not explicit: they exist as projections. If this projection of meaning is uncoupled from the ongoing dialogue, there is inhibition of each new shared moment of relationship, and the moment is separated out from past interpersonal experience.

Drew [121] illustrates how AIP can be used as an avoidance strategy and, for example, turns to the analysis of recordings of calls to a suicide-prevention hotline. Some callers avoid responding to a request for their name by turning the question back, that is, by asking the name of the clinician answering the phone (though a detour in conversation, the topic of identifying names is upheld). An interpolated silence, that is "not hearing" until the other party fills the conversation is another, potent avoidance strategy of AIP. A more elaborate avoidance strategy involves directing conversation to a similar topic, while not actually answering the question of the interviewer; for example, a question can be "answered" by another question which references the same subject (thus apparently supporting the sharing of a topic).

Avoidance strategies using AIP are not necessarily conscious, nor are they deliberately evasive. Their description demonstrates how expressive language – including verbal and nonverbal elements – can appear normal even while strict limits are imposed upon actual relationship. They suggest a mechanism rather than an etiology for disorders of attachment, one which entail social avoidance. As a dynamic process that unfolds over time, AIP is closer in meaning to attachment than is theory of mind. From the perspective of attachment theory, AIP provides an opportunity either to evade or to embrace the special connotations of shared experience that are founded upon the relational past.

Chapter 4
A Discussion and Critique of RAD

What Is Adaptive and What Is Pathology?

Findings of research and the theories for etiology of RAD present an apparent paradox: there is evidence of a genetic footprint, yet by definition a severely adverse environmental force is required at an early, critical stage of childhood. Gross neglect of an infant is inherently pathogenic for our species, in which the period of infant dependence is so prolonged. Neglect should decrease parental fitness, as measured by survival of offspring and this effect is magnified, not reduced, in situations of peril. Basic reflexes of our species (as in most mammals) serve to detect danger and to promote proximity of parent and infant, so that at speed, action comes first, reflection later. Powerful evolutionary pressure applies against abandonment because, compared to most species, the human infant has little chance for survival, without direct and close protection.

Despite this clear foundation for attachment in nature, there is recent critique of the premise that secure attachment is a normal condition, against which other forms of attachment can be contrasted or labeled as pathological. A key question is whether the human genome can support a host of attachment options, including the "best fit," to suboptimal conditions such as those of weak or even absent parental protection. Bjorklund and Pelligrini [122] summarize evidence against the premise that secure attachment is the norm, and they question the typology of the Strange Situation as overdetermined by the influence of Bowlby's theories. They observe that the majority of the American middle-class population first sampled is secure in attachment, but this is not true across cultures. For example, in a sample of Northern German infants, 49% met criteria for an avoidant attachment subtype; whereas only 33% met criteria for secure attachment [123]. In certain settings, secure attachment may even be deleterious; DeVries [124] reports that during a period of drought and famine, a tribe of Masai in Kenya lost 7 of 13 children, of which 5 had been identified as having "easy temperament." It appears that infants with easy temperament were at relative disadvantage compared to fussy or demanding infants during this cycle of hardship, as likely to be ignored, and hence to perish (though they received close parent support in times of plenty).

D.F. Shreeve, *Reactive Attachment Disorder: A Case-Based Approach,*
SpringerBriefs in Child Development, DOI 10.1007/978-1-4614-1647-0_4,
© Springer Science+Business Media, LLC 2012

Perhaps the most direct challenge to a dogma of secure attachment is a theory of Belsky et al. [125] according to which even in advanced technological societies, insecure attachment may convey relative advantage as measured in terms of biological fitness. The authors demonstrate that economic hardship correlates with early pubescence in girls as well as with family conflict, inconsistent parenting, father's absence, and lack of emotional support. In the hard light of evolutionary theory, emotional deprivation could theoretically favor endocrine changes in prepubescence which hasten reproductive maturity, in turn predisposing to early sexual behavior, as well as to short-lived relationships, which in turn promote early departure from home of origin. This would increase reproductive fitness if there is otherwise a low chance for material and emotional support from either biological parent.

Two alternative reproductive strategies are thus proposed by Belsky et al., each contingent upon resources and support. A secure attachment is favored for girls when there is high parental protection and ample resources: this strategy entails delay of puberty, with preparation for a subsequent long-lived pair bond supported by high investment in offspring by the protected daughters. In contrast, insecure attachment is adaptive to a social climate of transitory, superficial attachment, and resource scarcity. Reproductive fitness increases, according to the authors, as a consequence of early menarche, with priority of mating over rearing investment, essentially a reproductive strategy for affected families of "quantity over quality."

Belsky et al. provide a critique for their own theory for the phenomenon of early puberty in girls. A particular obstacle for a theory of stress-induced menarche is the phenomenon of anorexia nervosa: in this condition of frank starvation, menstruation ceases entirely. Although this would seem to present a contradiction, an alternative scenario can be imagined, possibly closer to ancestral history of *Homo sapiens*; this is the ancient human experience with cyclic shifts between abundance and starvation. Within this context, high stress at the beginning of the collapse of resources could trigger early maturation of females, who (unconsciously) capitalize on resources for reproduction just ahead of the period of famine, after which point natural selection favors a conservation strategy and inhibition of sexual development. Under these conditions those females with precocious puberty would have higher reproductive fitness, in comparison to girls who failed to respond hormonally to stress factors linked to changes in resource availability. For the parents of such girls, and since environmental shifts vary unpredictably, a variability of phenotype increases biological fitness so that some offspring at least survive in either condition of feast or famine to the time of reproduction. Variability in genetic expression, as observed by the authors, is also the raw material for the evolutionary process of natural selection.

The question of stress effect on age of puberty in boys receives little attention from the authors. Evolutionary pressures however, plausibly affect girls more because of their greater investment in reproductive effort (including care of the young). The authors propose that girls raised in a climate of stress are prone to internalizing symptoms such as depression and anxiety, "which serve to lower metabolism, store fat, and thereby stimulate menarche." In comparison, family hardship may favor externalizing symptoms for boys (though an evolutionary argument is not fully elaborated for this). For either gender, according to Belsky et al., early deprivation favors a kind of interpersonal opportunism, not consciously pursued but rather shaped by evolutionary pressure, in anticipation of environmental conditions which favor variably brief relationship. The theory of stress-induced early maturation is thus consistent with inter-generational effects of attachment disorder as costs of poverty and social alienation. These are seen repeatedly in the poverty cycle, as high rates of marital discord, child neglect, and abandonment.

Although the authors present a plausible explanation of insecure attachment as adaptive, this does not necessarily apply to actual absence of selective attachment, which is at the core of RAD, unless this deficit is interpreted as an extension of the identified trait for the capacity for transitory and facile attachment. Reactive attachment could theoretically arise in parallel with a greater readiness to actually abandon offspring: such a trait would, however, appear to violate evolutionary theory on the basis of the dramatic cost to maternal reproductive fitness. The classic work of Trivers [126] explains the differential parental investment of males and females, which begins with the greater cost of the ovum (measured in decrease in reproductive potential of other ova) and increases with each step of the reproductive process. For our species, and nearly all higher animals, female parental investment increases through the process of conception through birth and early rearing; this is a cumulative investment with compounding interest which reduces the reproductive advantage of abandonment by females virtually to zero. In evolutionary terms, readiness to abandon can increase reproductive fitness of males, who may be unsure of their own offspring and especially when they are generally able to mate again. In females of nearly all species, there can be no equivalent increase in reproductive fitness for a trait of "easy abandonment" because of cumulative, continuously accruing parental investment.

A separate explanation is possible for reactive attachment in epigenetic terms: fetal programming. Consider that an epigenetic adaptation to marginal subsistence in the primordial past could be maladaptive in modern, industrial culture, even deemed pathological. Neel's seminal theory of a "thrifty genotype" for diabetes [127] comprises an elegant example: a genetic predisposition for diabetes may be the vestige of an adaptation to feast and famine, in which context rapid rise in insulin would maximize energy stores when food becomes available. A tendency to hypoglycemia in some prediabetic children suggests just such high glucose efficiency at an early stage of diabetes after which insulin resistance (mediated by an unknown serum factor) produces hyperglycemia. As explained by Gluckman and Hanson [128], efficient metabolism of available nutrition is likely to have especially increased survivorship for under-weight, premature babies, but once "turned on" the genes for rapid weight gain convey high risk for insulin resistance, midlife diabetes, and heart disease.

Since the debt incurred for the thrifty gene is postponed until middle age, it is insulated from evolutionary pressure (since biological fitness is a function of rate of reproduction). Large-scale epidemiologic research supports the thrifty gene hypothesis in that the risk of adult cardiovascular illness is especially high for those born premature who continue to accelerate on the growth curve in the school-age period [129]. British epidemiologic research has also demonstrated a geographic distribution of diabetes that corresponds to poverty and unemployment, rather than to the affluence usually thought to predict diabetes [130]. If this model of a thrifty gene for high insulin is realistic, the central obesity of middle age actually is programmed before birth, and primary prevention of adult heart disease would require a greater focus on prenatal health!

Gluckman and Hanson extend the premise of the thrifty gene in their advance of general theory of Predictive Adaptive Response, according to which epigenetic programming is mediated by maternal physiology in order to optimize the fit of offspring to resource conditions at birth (either present, or in the ancestral past). An appeal of the model of fetal programming is that phenotypic shift is potentially much faster than the operation of natural selection on frequency of genotypes: its time span matches the shifts of resource changes in real time. The authors propose that, through the mediation of maternal physiological response to starvation or stress, the adaptation of offspring to resource scarcity may begin prior to birth.

Talge et al. [79] expound upon the model of Predictive Adaptive Response to explain a potential evolutionary basis for ADHD and take an example from nature (also mentioned in Gluckman and Hanson) to demonstrate fetal programming of behavioral phenotype. The case is that of the snowshoe hare of the Hudson Bay area. In this ecosystem, weather shifts drastically affect vegetation and periodically – roughly every 10 years – the population crashes, in turn precipitating an equal, but delayed, die-off of predators of the hare such as lynx and coyote. The net effect is that at its lowest population point, a generation of snowshoe hare is exposed to maximum predation pressure. It is this generation which must be continually on alert, for danger is ever-present. In behavioral terms, this generation of hares is essentially "born restless." Talge et al. conclude that "this type of fetal adaptive response to stressful surroundings has presumably developed in primates, including humans...extreme vigilance and rapid shifts in attention could be adaptive in an environment full of danger: in our modern culture, with no predators, extra vigilance and rapid shifts can be maladaptive, and can result in unnecessary anxiety and problems with attention."

To take this model of Predictive Adaptive Response from the snowshoe hare example one step further to an epigenetic mechanism of RAD might draw us onto the thin ice of open speculation. Yet we can apply the terms from Triver's theory of parental investment to derive necessary constraints for this theoretic application: a maternal stress effect which could impinge upon dyadic attachment would necessarily be extreme. Fetal programming to activate nonselective attachment would increase maternal biologic fitness only if the probability of the mother's own survival into the postnatal period is minimal, the necessary condition for even odds of survival when reared collectively by within a tribe. This pre-adapted mode would be induced by maternal stress effects, which program the fetus for subsequent, postnatal expression of particular attachment traits that carry relative advantage in a period of extreme hardship. Such a phenotype, in the evolutionary past, would maximize success through rapid but superficial attachment, and would be predisposed to vigilance as well as to early shift toward independence.

A discussion of potential adaptive advantage under extreme stress is of course inferential. We know only that genes may influence predisposition to RAD, and that pathogenic care causes RAD in some, but not all children exposed. The model of Predictive Adaptive Response illustrates how an epigenetic mechanism, generally involving a "fight or flight" predisposition, might arise early in the course of human history, and could persist in the modern day of generally abundant resources even if carrying risk for psychopathology.

The resilience of the many children who experience grossly pathogenic care is further evidence for the flexible range of human adaptation, expanding our definition of "normal." The recovery of many children from extreme symptoms, even from the appearance of apathy and "frozen watchfulness," is also proof that underlying brain structures for attachment may remain viable beyond critical periods of exposure, and may survive even the most extreme conditions of adversity.

Chapter 5
Therapy for RAD

Since psychotherapy is the primary treatment of RAD, the child psychiatrist seeks to provide this or to arrange a referral at the earliest opportunity. An obvious impediment to early success in child psychotherapy is the child's deficit in basic trust. Without trust, effectiveness of verbal therapy is particularly limited. The child's wish to please an adult is also normally a factor which mitigates the challenge of working on an unfamiliar project with a stranger. The process of therapy relies – at least in part – on a trust in the sharing of feelings, thoughts, and goals. When therapy is very slow or appears to stall, some clinicians and caregivers are inclined to specialized treatments, or "therapy by other means." This phenomenon can have the effect of sparking creative adaptations of child treatment, or conversely can serve as an apparent permission for treatments dominated by dogma and clinical lore.

Controversial techniques for treatment of RAD – also termed counterintuitive or paradoxical – can be divided into those which may be harmful, and those which are simply not yet empirically tested. Examples of techniques with poor evidence and high risk include forcefully hugging the child "until they are calm," restricting food or water, denying access to those outside the family, or rigidly demanding instant obedience to every command [27]. A particularly high-risk example is promoted as "re-birthing" – a process in which clinicians wrap the child in a blanket and hold tight until the child ceases to cry out. This intervention is known to have resulted in death [9], and hence is listed in the category of both potentially harmful and unsupported by evidence in the practice parameter of the American Academy of Child and Adolescent Psychiatry [26, 131].

In contrast is the clinical intervention termed "Theraplay" [132], a derivative of conventional play therapy which does sometimes employ touch, for example, in a game of "patty cake," or a make-believe face painting (with imaginary paints). Therapists are encouraged to "be delightful," to show excitement about the child, to share in the child's process of discovery, and to assist the child in mastery in creative play. While methods include the instruction to "use every opportunity to make physical contact with the child" this is for the purpose of modeling for the caregiver, who is present. Precaution against any semblance of inappropriate touch is likewise guided

D.F. Shreeve, *Reactive Attachment Disorder: A Case-Based Approach*,
SpringerBriefs in Child Development, DOI 10.1007/978-1-4614-1647-0_5,
© Springer Science+Business Media, LLC 2012

by the principle of attunement to the child's state of emotion, and by monitoring the child's capacity for stimulus load. Though touching can thus be a part of treatment, the techniques are essentially opposite to those of "forced holding" in that it is the child's purposes and intentions which come first in treatment.

The steps of Theraplay begin with careful observations of the child interacting with their parent figure and may include structured observations of the parent and child together. Based on the acquired perspective achieved through interacting with their caregiver, the therapist is ready to confidently guide parent and child into forms of play which maximize the child's enjoyment of mastery, and especially the opportunity to see wonder reflected in the eyes of the parent figure. Phases of structuring, nurturing, and challenging are individualized for the particular child, who is both subject and object of the process. Though therapists are taught to be confident leaders, they are also striving to be models for the parent figure: parent or foster parent is therefore an essential part of each session.

In general, other child therapies for RAD also prioritize the parent–child relationship, both in design of methods and in measurement of effect. Longer, more intensive therapies have been found to be superior at increasing parent sensitivity and enhancing children's attachment security [133]. In working with families of RAD children, the therapist seeks to identify defective parental response to understand its meaning and to facilitate alternative, new and satisfying ways of responding. In general, each of the accepted therapy methods helps the parent attune to the child and to combine sensitive understanding with correct setting of limits. Therefore, whether working with an adoptive family, or with parents who are overcoming a cycle of abuse, the initial goal of therapy is to strengthen attachment to a trusted caregiver. This may involve repair of reflexes shaped by the anticipation of rejection, and helping the caregiver to model new, mutually supportive relationship.

A further example of an effective therapy method is the Circle of Security Model [134], which aims to establish the parent as a zone of support and encouragement, thereby helping parent and child to formulate their relationship as positive and consistent. Infant-Parent Therapy and Child-Parent Therapy [135] are other potentially successful treatments which are based on the principal of enhancing relationship. Family therapy methods have also been systematically applied to RAD and may be useful in helping an adopted child integrate emotionally with new parent figures, and with new siblings [136].

An example of a repair intervention with little established proof but with low risk is the recent therapy tool of "Time In." Purvis et al. [137] advise parents of attachment disorder children to draw close to their child after an incident of bad behavior, rather than punishing them with the conventional "time out." This may repair the negative self-image which has accrued from too many repetitions of "time out," an experience of physical isolation that has come to symbolize rejection. When the parent maintains proximity through the course of and episode of shame and felt rejection, a repair occurs which inclines the child to trust in adult guidance and protection.

An essential part of effective attachment therapy is preparation for the emergence of post-traumatic symptoms. These may emerge unevenly, sometimes unexpectedly, as the child increasingly begins to employ reflection in place of defensive reflexes.

Trauma effects may for example surface in the form of a rise in oppositional-defiant disorder [138]. Children exposed to repeated trauma may show a combination of post-traumatic symptoms, deficits in self-regulation of emotions, and attachment problems. Therapy for such complex trauma disorder emphasizes development of a sense of safety, and strives to replace defensive emotional reactions to trauma memories with coping strategies [111, 112]. Personal engagement, exploration of self-assertion, and demonstration of reciprocity are key elements of this treatment. Capacity for self-regulation of emotions, presumed to be damaged by trauma, is enhanced through reliance on the therapeutic relationship and direct practice with self-calming (coping) strategies. In a review of the "Attachment, Self-Regulation, and Competency (ARC)" model, Kinniburgh [111] observe that "ARC highlights attachment as a primary domain of intervention and focuses on two overarching goals for attachment-focused interventions: building healthy attachments between those children who have experienced trauma and their caregivers; and creating the safe environment for healthy recovery that has been affected by the trauma or was largely absent even before."

It should also be remembered that the child psychiatry clinician joins with other child providers to make a team, the purpose of which is to ensure that the affected child is assigned to a trustworthy family, and that a worthy assignment of care has every chance to succeed. Maintaining an active and flexible membership on the treatment team is therefore a guiding principal for psychiatry. From a background of defects in attachment, comorbid conditions emerge, sometimes unpredictably, which require an available and responsive psychiatry clinician. Anxiety, depression, attention deficit disorder, conduct and impulse problems are examples of comorbidity, which may benefit from psychiatry medication treatment. Case managers, therapist, and families also want the psychiatrist to assist in prioritizing symptoms, and in formulating a treatment plan which is based on a developmental perspective.

The inherent difficulty of working with damage to basic trust is that progress may be slow, sometimes painstaking. Episodes of regression – or setbacks in the treatment plan – typically involve multiple symptom domains and sometimes cast into doubt as to whether any progress is made at all. Cooperative teamwork is the solution to doubts about the direction of care, as it is so often our human solution to challenging circumstance. When individual skills are applied collectively, confidence is engendered through teamwork, is shared with the family, and becomes therapeutic for the child with RAD. Challenges in treatment are compensated – in many cases – by the opportunity to witness a remarkable unfolding of the human capacity for intimate and enduring attachment.

Test #2: Theory Questions

1. Which of the following is the best example of an attachment behavior as defined by Bowlby?

(a) A 3-year-old gets lost from his mother in a grocery store, and his noisy cries persist even though the storeowner and security personnel do everything possible to reassure him.

(b) At his first session with you, a 5-year-old smiles at you and tries to give a full bear hug.

(c) A 7-year-old tries to follow the mailman on his rounds and asks if he can join the postal service.

(d) A teenager posts her photograph and a description of herself on an Internet site, inviting other teenagers to share interests.

(e) A 5-year-old is lost in the park but stops crying when he sees a policeman.

2. Which of the following is typically the most persistent over time in a child with RAD and no other diagnosis who is transferred to a stable environment?

(a) General delays in expressive speech.

(b) Indiscriminate friendliness

(c) Quasi-autistic symptoms which resemble features of autism

(d) Freezing at the sight of an adult approaching and refusing or declining to interact

(e) Inappropriate and sexualized behavior toward younger children

3. Which group of researchers discovered that on administration of a test of separation and reunion, even securely attached children may briefly avoid eye contact or interaction with their parent figure upon their return?

(a) Ainsworth

(b) Main and Weston

(c) Bowlby

(d) Lewis

(e) Schore

4. Which of the following is an example of a displacement activity occurring in a young child during moments of separation anxiety?

(a) The child shows rapid shifts in approach and withdrawal upon the reunion phase of the Strange Situation test.

(b) The child avoids eye contact with the parent upon reunion and moves away when they approach.

(c) The child threatens another child in the waiting area who steps between him and his mother.

(d) The child wants to wander off with a stranger as soon as his mother leaves the room.

(e) The child appears to busy himself building a tower with blocks when his mother comes back in the room.

5. The theory that grossly pathogenic care in early childhood leads to actual atrophy or permanent maldevelopment of limbic networks is best attributed to:

(a) Schore

(b) Joseph

(c) Lewis

(d) Siegel

(e) Cassidy

B. Matching Section

Match the following by inserting the appropriate letter next to the corresponding social or psychological process (use each letter once):

_____ 6. Theory of Mind

_____ 7. Anticipatory Interactive Planning

_____ 8. Machiavellian Intelligence

_____ 9. Alexithymia

_____ 10. Indiscriminate Friendliness

(a) Gail's expression worries her friend Julie, as they sit down for a break during a shopping trip. She pats Gail's hand and asks her whether she has found everything she was hoping to find while they were shopping together.

(b) A college student enters the subway and strikes up a conversation about guitars with a man carrying a guitar case.

(c) A political official spreads the word that competition is keen for a committee over which he presides. The committee has yet to convene or to establish an agenda, but he expects that competition will sort out who is most closely allied with him, while at the same his prestige will increase as a function of the competition for membership.

(d) A 12-year-old newly admitted to inpatient psychiatry is asked why he has cut his arm superficially with a pocket knife on the day of admission, and he responds by saying that "it must mean that he was feeling suicidal."

(e) Perceiving that his friend Jay has paused awkwardly when the conversation turns to the subject of family life, Tom steers the conversation to the topic of favorite TV sports programs.

Appendix A
Answer Key for Case-Related Questions

1. The correct answer is: **c**
   a. *Incorrect.* There is no research evidence favoring administration of growth hormone for purpose of improving self-esteem in children with growth retardation secondary to neglect, and even with evidence this would not be an initial intervention.
   b. *Incorrect.* If norms for size are different in Guatemala, this does not mean that delay in growth is not a particular problem for Jorge, and there is no comparative information provided which would dismiss the importance of a pediatric consult.
   c. *Correct.* Early pediatric or family medication evaluation is important based on the high rate of health concerns in international adoptees, which include delays of vaccinations, in addition to growth problems and other pediatric problems.
   d. *Incorrect.* Postponing care on the basis of missing records aggravates and compounds the problem of past medical neglect.
   e. *Incorrect.* Supporting a "wait-and-see" approach may reinforce a false optimism, and could result in missing an important medical problem.

2. The correct answer is: **c**
   a. *Incorrect.* Collaborative treatment is essential for RAD, and Jorge will benefit from close liaison between specialties. Consent for shared discussion is a task often best completed at intake.
   b. *Incorrect.* Exclusively restricting psychiatry to medication managements diminishes your usefulness to the treatment team.
   c. *Correct.* Symptoms evolve over time in RAD, sometimes as new developmental tasks are encountered, or as a function of stress. A continuing membership on the team is helpful in meeting the variable challenges of treatment care. Ongoing availability also means that medication trials do not extend beyond their useful purpose.
   d. *Incorrect.* You will not be accepted on the team with this approach.

D.F. Shreeve, *Reactive Attachment Disorder: A Case-Based Approach*,
SpringerBriefs in Child Development, DOI 10.1007/978-1-4614-1647-0,
© Springer Science+Business Media, LLC 2012

e. *Incorrect.* It is hazardous to recommend advanced treatments without knowing about the methods you will appear to have endorsed. Advanced methods such as forced holds and re-birthing have caused significant harm.

3. The correct answer is: **a**
   a. *Correct.* Gathering information about symptoms from two or more settings is a standard part of the evaluation for ADHD. This step does not necessarily lead to diagnosis or treatment, and it will be important to know if the symptoms are limited to specific contexts, supporting the therapist's view. If Jorge has ADHD symptoms in multiple settings, he may benefit from treatment of this comorbid condition.
   b. *Incorrect.* There is no evidence of paradoxical effect of medication treatment for ADHD in children with both RAD and ADHD.
   c. *Incorrect.* There is actually less reason to send Jorge to residential treatment at the point of suspecting that ADHD is a part of his symptom picture. His general adaptation may improve if ADHD is correctly diagnosed and treated.
   d. *Incorrect.* With the information provided, there is no rationale for either brain imaging or genetic testing at this point, and neither is standard of care in the initial assessment of ADHD symptoms.
   e. *Incorrect.* There is no evidence provided which suggests that Jorge has a limitation in language that affects therapy. Interrupting therapy also presents a risk for Jorge, who is gradually establishing a capacity for trust and selective relationship.

4. The correct answer is: **a**
   a. *Correct.* To address the problem behavior it is important to know what Jorge has learned about the touch behavior, what it means to him, and what he understands to be the effect on others. Cultural differences, if any, would also apply to evaluating the behavior, and comprehending the motivation of the behavior is a first step in addressing treatment.
   b. *Incorrect.* Simply assigning time in the corner does not help Jorge to clarify his own motivations, and this peremptory adult response is likely to reinforce his behavioral reactions to past emotional neglect.
   c. *Incorrect.* Simulating an incorrect social behavior is contraindicated, as it is likely to confuse a child like Jorge, and will interfere with the acquisition of social norms.
   d. *Incorrect.* Although lack of reinforcement could plausibly lead to extinction of a behavior, it will activate Jorge's envy of the other children and resentment which relates to unmet dependency need. Without interpreting the meaning of turning away, his teacher will likely see a rise in oppositional-defiant behavior.
   e. *Incorrect.* Not addressing the social cost of an inappropriate behavior is counterintuitive and will interfere with Jorge's acquisition of social norms. As he becomes self-conscious of the adult effort to avoid criticism, he is likely to internalize a negative self-image.

5. The correct answer is: **d**
   a. *Incorrect.* An age-appropriate, developmental task for Jorge is to distinguish between having feelings of anger and behaving aggressively. Apologizing for the appearance of feeling angry will thwart him in his effort to cope with angry feelings within socially acceptable ways, such as explaining rather than "acting out" feelings.
   b. *Incorrect.* While unconditional affection plays an important role in early dyadic attachment, providing this in a broader social context would foster a false and unrealistic expectation of his relationship to school.
   c. *Incorrect.* Though the sanction of expulsion may be explained calmly this does not represent object constancy, as it is in fact retaliatory.
   d. *Correct.* Although object constancy originally applied to the maintenance of an internalized image of the parent independent of drive states, it now applies also to modeling of calm, predictable response to provocation by the responsible parent or adult figure. Here the therapist represents object constancy by calmly explaining rules that comprise a structure for social adaptation.
   e. *Incorrect.* Assigning all social correction to a parent is unrealistic, as social crises require resolution in the moment they occur. Hinting that forceful punishment is permissible outside the school is irresponsible.

6. The correct answer is: **b**
   a. *Incorrect.* Although weight gain may be an unfortunate side effect, a 2-week washout on the inpatient unit is costly, and may be unproductive. If effective, the current mood stabilizer may need to be continued while alternatives are considered, hopefully with a better side effect profile.
   b. *Correct.* Although you are not directing inpatient treatment and may not have all the facts, it is important to know whether there is any chance that the start of an antidepressant might have aggravated the current behavioral symptoms. It is not unusual for antidepressants to be started with the theory that external symptoms represent a masked depression: sometimes this is correct, and at other times discontinuing an antidepressant may significantly improve the level of symptoms.
   c. *Incorrect.* A portion of RAD children may worsen time in a structured setting, and within the close quarters of an inpatient milieu. The inpatient team is familiar with the current symptoms, and therefore has a better perspective as to whether residential treatment is required.
   d. *Incorrect.* Recommendation of removal from the home and transfer is hazardous, as it will likely impair or destroy your treatment alliance with the Smiths if they disagree. The inpatient team will then need to hunt for a new child psychiatrist.
   e. *Incorrect.* You cannot guide the inpatient medication plan since you are not the current treating physician.

7. The correct answer is: **d**
   a. *Incorrect*. Reactivation of trauma is a risk of therapy, and management of the affect aroused by recovered memory is a part of the skill set for therapists who work with childhood trauma.
   b. *Incorrect*. Coercive treatments have a proven risk in the treatment of RAD.
   c. *Incorrect*. Medication treatment options are not well defined for childhood PTSD, and the risk of discontinuing other treatments for such a medication trial is high relative to benefit. Of note, an off-label medication trial might be considered if trauma symptoms are chronically severe. At this point, the rise in symptoms is acute and evidently reactive to a single session of therapy.
   d. *Correct*. Encouragement of the current therapy treatment alliance will help Jorge to become confidant about managing negative emotions and will likely further his trust in how adults work together to manage problems. Checking with the therapist about treatment could be useful if this is a new colleague, so as to politely verify an understanding of the methods in use.
   e. *Incorrect*. Nightmares are common in PTSD, and at this point there is no information to suggest a primary sleep disorder.

8. The correct answer is: **c**
   a. *Incorrect*. As described in the text, a minority of RAD children show persistence of quasi-autistic symptoms, that improve over time. In this case autistic symptoms are becoming increasingly severe.
   b. *Incorrect*. It is rare to see autistic symptoms persist unchanged in the inhibited-withdrawn type of RAD, and this form of RAD is typically responsive to placement in a supportive environment.
   c. *Correct*. As listed in the DSMIV, diagnosis is made for ASD when full criteria are met, even when attachment disorder affects the capacity for interpersonal relatedness.
   d. *Incorrect*. It is the disinhibited form of RAD which shows greater persistence of symptoms, as manifest, for example, in excessive friendliness to strangers.
   e. *Incorrect*. The rage behavior so far described relates to insistence on sameness, an autistic trait. Unless further history is provided about episodic mood changes, there is no present basis for diagnosis of bipolar disorder.

9. The correct answer is: **b**
   a. *Incorrect*. The extent and duration of tantrum behavior after reunion does not match with secure attachment.
   b. *Correct*. Timmy is showing shifts between approach and withdrawal behavior, while maintaining the high emotional intensity characteristic of disorganized attachment.
   c. *Incorrect*. Intense emotional display exclusively directed to the parent figure practically rules out RAD.

d. *Incorrect.* Although play behavior may have helpfully distracted Timmy from his separation anxiety, the severity and duration of rage after reunion does not match with secure attachment.

e. *Incorrect.* Timmy is rather persistent and tenacious in his expression of anger, which therefore does not seem like an impulsive mistake. The reunion behavior is in any case not a proof for ADHD, which therefore cannot be invoked to explain the intense, ambivalent display of anger toward his mother.

10. The correct answer is: **c**

a. *Incorrect.* A substituted gesture, following Winnicott, would not take account of the child's motivation or would oppose the direction of an intention.

b. *Incorrect.* Pseudomaturity refers to the assumption of a false or artificial level of independence and precocious manner.

c. *Correct.* By helping to overcome an obstacle and furthering an original intention, there is recognition of the child's aims and an empathic identification with the child's sense of agency.

d. *Incorrect.* After providing helpful assistance, this parent allows the child to independently further their original goal.

e. *Incorrect.* The parent is evidently aware that her child is startled by the mishap. Though it is understandable that other adults in the waiting area might be irked, the mother's attunement inclines her to show that the accident is a problem that can be fixed.

Appendix B
Answer Key for Theory Questions

1. The correct answer is: **a**
   a. Crying is an attachment behavior, and selective attachment is suggested by the worsening of behavior when a stranger urges the child to desist.
   b. A warm smile and a hug by an unaccompanied 5-year-old just meeting you suggest a potential problem of attachment, and in any case the behaviors do not represent normal attachment.
   c. The strong interest in a stranger is not biological attachment as described by Bowlby; further context is needed to clarify the meaning of the behavior.
   d. Posting on the internet to strangers is almost the opposite of attachment.
   e. The meaning is unclear, but the cessation of crying at the sight of an officer is not an attachment behavior.

2. The correct answer is: **b**
   For choices a–d, the most persistent RAD symptom is indiscriminate friendliness (b). Sexualized behavior in childhood PTSD has variable persistence, but is not specifically part of RAD criteria.

3. The correct answer is: **b**
   Main and Weston continued the work of Ainsworth and confirmed many of the original findings, but disputed the observation that avoidance of engagement at point of reunion necessarily reveals insecure attachment; brief avoidance of eye contact, for example, also occurs in some children who are securely attached.

4. The correct answer is: **e**
   a. The behaviors show rapid shifts between conflicting intentions, suggesting disorganized attachment.
   b. Avoidance and anxiety is depicted, rather than displacement of arousal into an apparently unrelated activity.
   c. The child's behavior corresponds closely to the represented goal of preserving access to the parent.
   d. Indiscriminate friendliness is represented.

e. This displacement activity allows time for dissipation of a portion of highly charged emotions, and after a brief moment the child may be able to reengage without showing negative affect.

5. The correct answer is: **b**

While multiple authors have theorized that early deficits in attachment impair the development of limbic networks, only Joseph compares early deprivation to actual ablation experiments in animals.

6–10.   The correct answers are:

6. **a**

Julie interprets Gail's state of mind based on shared experience, as well as an appreciation of Gail's individual perspective.

7. **e**

Tom redirects to a topic which he estimates Jay will share, thus extending the opportunity for interaction.

8. **c**

This official reflects on the motivations of his staff and uses the information from his human study to advance a personal agenda.

9. **d**

This pre-adolescent appears to be repeating what he has been told about his own state of mind, rather than revealing emotion.

10. **b**

The teenager displays a nondiscriminate social drive and neglects to consider the other passenger's possible objection to interaction in the crowded setting.

References

1. Ainsworth, M.D.S., and Bell, S.M. (1970). Attachment, exploration, and separation: illustrated by the behavior of one-year-olds in a strange situation. Child Developm, 41 (1): 49–67.
2. Bowlby, J. (1982). Attachment and Loss, Vol 1:Attachment. Basic Books, New York.
3. Main, M. (1996). Introduction to the special section on attachment and psychopathology: overview of the field of attachment. J Cons Clinical Psychol, 64 (2): 237–243.
4. Ainsworth, M.D.S., Belhar, M.S., Waters, E. and Wall, S. (1978). Patterns of Attachment: A Psychological Study of the Strange Situation. Hillsdale, N.J.: Erlbaum.
5. Main, M., and Solomon, J. (1990). Procedures for identifying infants as disorganized/disoriented during the Ainsworth strange situation. **In**: M.T. Greenberg, D. Cicchetti, and E.M. Cummings (Eds.) Attachment in the Preschool Years: Theory, research, and interventions (pp. 121–160). Chicago: University of Chicago Press.
6. Mahler, M.S., Pine, F., and Bergman, A. (1975). The Psychological Birth of the Human Infant: Symbiosis and Individuation.New York: Basic Books.
7. Pine, F. (2004). Mahler's concepts of "symbiosis" and separation-individuation: Revisited, re-evaluated, and refined. J Am Psychoanal Assoc, 52 (2): 511–533.
8. Winnicott, D.W. (1960). The Maturational Process and the Facilitating Environment: Studies in the Theory of Emotional Development. New York: International Universities Press.
9. Shreeve, D.F. (1990). Pseudomaturity in the developmental line of object relations. Am J Psychother, 24(4): 536–551.
10. Stern, D. (1985). The Interpersonal World of the Human Infant: A View from Psychoanalysis and Developmental Psychology. New York: Basic Books.
11. Stern, D.W., Hoffer, L., Haft, W., and Dore, J. (1987). L'accordage affectif; Le partage d'états émotionnels entre mère et enfant par écharges sur un mode croise. Annale S Médico Psychologiques, 145(3): 205–224.
12. Tronick, E. (1989). Emotions and emotional communication in infants. Am Psychologist, 44(2): 112–119.
13. Emde, R.N., Kligmar, D.H., Reich, J.H., and Wade, T.D. (1978). Emotional expression in infancy: Initial studies of social signaling and an emergent model. In M. Lewis and L.A. Rosenblum (Eds.), The Development of Affect (pp. 125–148). New York: Plenum Press.
14. Trevarthen, C. (1979). Communication and cooperation in early infancy: A description of primary intersubjectivity. **In** M.M. Bullowa (Ed.), Before Speech: The Beginning of Interpersonal Communication (pp. 321–349). New York: Cambridge University Press.
15. Trevarthen, C. (1980). The foundations of intersubjectivity: Development of interpersonal and cooperative understanding in infants. **In** D. Olsen (Ed.), The Social Foundations of Language and Thought: Essays in Honor of J.S. Bruner (pp. 316–342). New York: Norton.

16. Van Egeren, L.A.; Barratt, M.S., and Roach, M.A. (2001). Mother-infant responsiveness: Timing, mutual regulation, and interactional context. Developm Psychol, 37 (5): 684–697.

17. Cassidy, J. (1994). Emotions regulation: Influences of attachment relationships. MonSoc Res Child Developm 59 (2–3): 228–249.

18. Vygotsky, L.S. (1978). Mind in Society: The Development of Higher Psychological Processes. Cambridge: Harvard University Press.

19. Diagnostic and Statistical Manual, 4th Edition (2000). New York: American Psychiatric Association.

20. Solomon, J. and George, C. (1999). The measurement of attachment security in infancy and childhood. In J. Cassidy, and P.R. Shaver (Eds.), Handbook of Attachment: Theory, Research, and Clinical Applications(pp. 287–318). Guilford Press, New York.

21. Minnis, H., Rabe-Hesketh, S., and Wolkind, S. (2001). Development of a brief, clinically relevant, scale for measuring attachment disorders. J Meth Psychiatric Res, 11(2): 90–98.

22. Rutter, M., Anderson-Wood, L, Beckett, C., et al, and the English and Romanian Adoptees (ERA) Study Team (1999). Quasi-autistic patterns following severe early global privation. J ChildPsychol Psychiatry, 40:537–549.

23. Franc, N., Maury, M., and Purper-Oaukil, D. (2009). Trouble déficit de l'attention/hyperactivité: quel lien avec l'attachement.L'Encéphale, 35(3): 256–261.

24. Hall, S.E. and Geher, G. (2003). Behavioral and personality characteristics of children with Reactive Attachment Disorder. J Psychol, 137(2): 145–162.

25. Achenbach, T.M.,and Rescorla, L.A. (2001). Manual for the ASEBA School-Age Forms and Profiles. Burlington, Vermont: University of Vermont Department of Psychiatry.

26. American Academy of Child and Adolescent Psychiatry (2005).Practice Parameter: Reactive Attachment Disorder.J Am Acad Child Adolesc Psychiatry, 44(11): 1206–1219.

27. Chaffin, M. et al (2006). Report of the APSAC Task Force on Attachment Therapy, Reactive Attachment Disorder, and Attachment Problems. Child Maltreat, 11(1): 76–89.

28. Achenbach, T.M., and Rescorla, L.A. (2000). Manual for the ASEBA Preschool Forms and Profiles. Burlington, Vermont: University of Vermont Department of Psychiatry.

29. Seabrook, J. (2010). The last babylift: Adopting a child in Haiti. New Yorker, May 2010 Issue:pp. 1–10.

30. Seabrook, J. (2010). The Joys and Struggles of International Adoption. NPR Telecast, May 14 (2010).

31. Bruce, J., Tarullo, A.R., and Gunnar, M.R. (2009). Disinhibited social behavior among internationally adopted children. DevelpmPsychopath, 21: 157–171.

32. Dubinsky, K. (2007). Babies without borders: Rescue, kidnap, and the symbolic child. J. Women's His, 29 (1): 142–150.

33. Kim, W.J. (1995). International adoption: A case review of Korean children. Child Psychiatry Hum Developm, 25 (3): 141–154.

34. Zeanah, C.H., and Boris, N.W. (2000). Disturbances and disorders of attachment in early childhood. In C.H. Zeanah (Ed.), Handbook of Infant Mental Health, 2nd Edition (Chpt. 22: 353–368). New York:Guilford Press.

35. Mitchell, W.G., Gorrell, R.W., and Greenberg, R.A. (1980). Failure-to-thrive: A study in a primary care setting, epidemiology and follow-up. Ped, 65(5): 971–977.

36. Casey, P.H., and Arnold, W.C. (1985). Compensatory growth in infants with severe failure to thrive. S Med J, 78(9): 1057–1060.

37. Chatoor, I., et al (1998). Attachment and feeding problems: A re-examination of nonorganic failure to thrive and attachment insecurity. J of the Am Acad Child and Adolesc Psychiatry, 37 (11): 1217–1224.

38. Miller, L. Chan, W., Comfort, K., and Tirella, L. (2005). Health of children adopted from Guatemala: Comparison of orphanage and foster Care. Ped, 115; e710-e717.

39. Famularo, R., Kinscherff, R., and Fenton, J. (1992). Psychiatric diagnoses of maltreated children: Preliminary findings. J Am Acad Child Adolesc Psychiatry, 31(5): 863–867.

40. Sund, A.M., and Wichstrom, L. (2002). Insecure attachment and future depression. J Am Acad Child Adolesc Psychiatry, 41(12): 1470–1478.

41. Scopler, E., Reichler, R.J., and Renner, B.R. (1999). CARS: The Childhood Autism Rating Scale. Los Angeles: Western Psychological Services.

42. Stoecker, T.J. (2010). Personal communication.Roanoke: Department of Radiology, Carilion Clinic.

43. Nimkin, K., Spevak, M.R., and Kleinman, P.K. (1997). Fractures of the hands and feet in child abuse: imaging and pathological features. Rad, 203: 233–237.

44. Kleinman, P.K., and Marks, S.C., Jr (1996). A regional approach to the classic metaphyseal lesion in abused infants: the proximal tibia. AJR, 166: 421–426.

45. Garcia, V.F., Gotschall, C.S., Eichelberger, M.R., and Bowman, L.M. (1990). Rib fractures in children: A marker of severe trauma. J Trauma, 30(6): 695–700.

46. Seltzer, L.J., Ziegler, T.E., and Pollak, S.D. (2010). Social vocalizations can release oxytocin in humans. Proc R Soc B, 227: 2661–2666.

47. Shreeve, D. F. (1991). Elective mutism: Origins in stranger anxiety and selective attention. Bul Menninger Clin, 55(4): 491–504.

48. Lemche, E., Klann-Delius, G., Koch, R., and Joraschky, P. (2004). Mentalizing language development in a longitudinal attachment sample: Implications for alexithymia. Psychother Psychosom, 73: 366–374.

49. Sifneos, P.E. (1973). The prevalence of alexithymic characteristics in psychosomatic patients. Psychother and Psychosom, 22: 255–262.

50. Way, I., Yelsma, P., Van Meter, A.M., and Black-Pond, C. (2007). Understanding alexithymia and language skills in children: Implications for assessment and intervention. Lang, Speech, Hear Serv Schools, 38: 128–139.

51. Lochman, J.E., and Dodge, K.A. (1994). Social-cognitive processes of severely violent, moderately aggressive, and non-aggressive boys. J Cons and Clin Psychol, 62 (2): 366–374.

52. Zadeh, Z.Y., Im-Bolter, N. and Cohen, N.J. (2007). Social cognition and externalizing psychopathology: An investigation of the mediating role of language. J Abnorm Child Psychol, 35 : 141–152.

53. Camras, L.A., Ribordy, S., Hill, J., Martino, S., et al (1990). Maternal facial behavior and the recognition of emotion expression by maltreated and nonmaltreated children. Developm Psychol, 26 (2): 304–312.

54. Wismer Fries, A.B., and Pollak, S.D. (2004). Emotion understanding in postinstitutionalized Eastern European children. Developm Psychopath, 16: 355–369.

55. Geller, E., and Foley, G.M. (2009). Expanding the "ports of entry" for speech-language pathologists: A relational and reflective model for clinical practice. A J Speech-Lang Path, 18: 4–21.

56. Hinshaw-Fuselier, S., Boris, N.W., and Zeanah, C.H. (1999). Reactive Attachment Disorder in maltreated twins. Infant Ment Health J, 20(1): 42–59.

57. Heller, S.S., Boris, N.W., Fuselier, S-H, et al (2006). Reactive Attachment Disorder in maltreated twins follow-up; From 18 months to 8 years. Attach Hum Developm; 8(1): 63–86

58. Tizard, B. and Rees, J. (1975). The effect of early institutional rearing on the behaviour problems and affectional relationships of four-year-old children. J Child Psychol Psychiatry, 16: 61–73.

59. Tizard, B. and Hodges, J. (1978). The effect of early institutional rearing on the development of eight-year-old children. J Child Psychol Psychiatry, 19: 99–118.

60. Hodges, J., and Tizard, B. (1989). Social and family relationships of ex-institutional adolescents. J Child Psychol Psychiatry, 30 (1): 77–97.

61. Rutter, M., Colvert, E., Kreppner, J., Croft, C., et al (2007). Early adolescent outcomes for institutionally-deprived and non-deprived adoptees. I: Disinhibited attachment. J Child Psychol Psychiatry, 48: 17–30.

62. Chisholm, K., Carter, M.C., and Ames, E.W., et al (1995). Attachment security and indiscriminately friendly behavior in children adopted from Romanian orphanages. Developm Psychopath, 7:283–298.

63. Lyons-Ruth, K., Bureau, J-F., Riley, C.D, and Atlas-Corbett, A. F. (2009). Socially indiscriminate attachment behavior in the strange situation: Convergent and discriminate validity

in relation to caregiving risk, later behavior problems, and attachment insecurity. Developm Psychopath, 21: 355–367.

64. Pears, K.C., Bruce, J. and Fisher, P.A. and Kim, H.K. (2009). Indiscriminate friendliness in maltreated foster children. Child Maltreat, 15 (1): 64–75.

65. Chisholm, K. (1998). A three-year follow-up of attachment and indiscriminate friendliness in children adopted from Romanian orphanages. Child Developm, 69 (4): 1092–1106.

66. O'Connor, T.G., Bredenkamp, D., Rutter, M., and the English and Romanian Adoptees (ERA) Study Team (1999). Attachment disturbances and disorders in children exposed to early severe deprivation. Infant Ment Health J, 20 (1): 10–29.

67. Zeanah, C.H., Smyke, A.T., and Dumitrescu, A. (2002). Disturbances of attachment in young children, II: Indiscriminate behavior and institutional care. J. Am. Child Adolesc Psychiatry, 41 (8): 983–989.

68. Cameron, C. A., Ungar, M., and Liebenberg, L. (2007). Cultural understandings of resilience: roots for wings in the development of affective resources for resilience. Child Adolesc Psychiatric Clin N Am, 16: 285–301.

69. Finkel, D., and Matheny, A.P. (2000). Genetic and environmental influences on a measure of infant attachment security. Twin Res, 3: 242–250.

70. Gervai, J., Nemoda, Z, Lakatos, K., et al. (2005). Transmission disequilibrium tests confirm the link between DRDF gene polymorphism and infant attachment. Am J Med Gen, 132B: 126–130.

71. Faraone, S.V., Doyle, A.E., Mick, E., and Biederman, J. (2001). Meta-analysis of the association between the 7-repeat allele of the dopamine D4 receptor gene and attention deficit hyperactivity disorder. Am J Psychiatry, 158: 1052–1057.

72. Claussen, A.H., Mundy, P.C., Mallik, S.A., and Willoughby, J.C. (2002). Joint attention and disorganized attachment status in infants at risk. Developm Psychopath, 14: 279–291.

73. Weaver, I.C.G., Cervoni, N., Champagne, F. A., et al (2004). Epigenetic programming by maternal behavior. Nat Neurosci, 7 (8): 847–854.

74. Zhang, T-Y., Parent, C., Weaver, I., and Meaney, M.J. (2004). Maternal programming of individual differences in defensive responses in the rat. Ann NY Acad Sci, 1032: 85–103.

75. Bagot, R.C., and Meaney, M.J. (2010). Epigenetics and the biological basis of gene x environment interactions. J Am Acad Child Adolesc Psychiatry, 49 (8): 752–771.

76. Lakatos, K., Toth, I., Nemoda, Z., et al (2000). Dopamine D4 (DRD4) gene polymorphism is associated with attachment disorganization in infants. Mole Psychiatry, 5: 633–637.

77. Spangler, G., Johann, M., Roani, Z., and Zimmerman, P. (2009). Genetic and environmental influences on attachment disorganization. J Child Psychol Psychiatry, 50(8): 952–961.

78. Walker, C-D, Deschamps, S., Proulx, K., et al. (2004). Mother to infant or infant to mother?: Reciprocal regulation of responsiveness to stress in rodents and the implication for humans. J PsychiatryNeurosci, 29 (5): 364–382.

79. Talge, N.M., Neal, C., Glover, V., and the Early Stress, Translational Research and Prevention Network: Fetal and Neonatal Experience on Child and Adolescent Mental Health(2007). Antenatal maternal stress and long-term effects on child neurodevelopment: how and why? J Child Psychol Psychiatry, 48 (3/4): 245–261.

80. Martins, C., and Gaffan, E.A. (2000). Effects of early maternal depression on patterns of infant-mother attachment: A meta-analytic investigation. J Child Psychol Psychiatry, 41 (6): 737–746.

81. Cogill, S.R., Caplan, H.L, Alexandra, H., et al (1986). Impacts of maternal post-natal depression on cognitive development of young children. Br Med J, 292: 1165–1167.

82. Murray, L, and Cooper, P. (1996). The impact of postpartum depression on child development. Int RevPsychiatry, 8: 55–63.

83. Shaw, D.S., and Vondra, J.I. (1995). Infant attachment security and maternal predictors of early behavior problems: A longitudinal study of low-income families. J Abnormal Child Psychol, 23 (3): 335–357.

84. Beeghly, M., Frank, D.A., Rose-Jacobs, R., et al (2003). Level of prenatal cocaine exposure and infant-caregiver attachment behavior. Neurotoxicol Teratol, 25: 22–38.

85. Joseph, R. (1999). Environmental influences on neural plasticity, the limbic system, emotional development and attachment: A review. Child Psychiatry Hum Developm, 29 (3): 189–206.

86. Harlow, H.F., and Harlow, M.K. (1969). Effects of various mother-infant relationships on rhesus monkey behaviours. In B.M. Foss (Ed.). Determinants of Infant Behaviour, Vol. 4 (pp. 15–36). London: Metheun,

87. Kling, A. (1972). Effects of amygdalectomy on social-affective behavior in non-human primates. In The Neurobiology of the Amygdale. B.E. Eleftherious (Ed.). New York: Plenum.

88. Schore, A.N. (2003). Affect Dysregulation and Disorders of the Self. New York:Norton and Company.

89. Schore, A.N. (2002). Dysregulation of the right brain: A fundamental mechanism of traumatic attachment and the psychopathogenesis of posttraumatic stress disorder. Aust NZ J Psychiatry, 36: 9–30.

90. Teicher, M.H., Andersen, S.L, Polcari, A., et al (2002). Developmental neurobiology of childhood stress and trauma. Psychiatr Clin N Am, 25: 397–426.

91. Van der Kolk, B.A., and Saporta, J. (1991). The biological response to psychic trauma: Mechanisms and treatment of intrusion and numbing. Anx Res (U.K.), 4: 199–212.

92. Oosterman, M. and Schuengel, C. (2007). Autonomic reactivity to separation and reunion with foster parents. J Am Acad Child Adolesc Psychiatry, 46: 1196–1203.

93. Ahnert, L., Gunnar, M.R., Lamb, M.E., and Barthel, M. (2004). Transition to child care: Associations with infant-mother attachment, infant negative emotion, and cortisol elevations. Child Developm, 75 (3): 639–650.

94. Spangler, G., and Grossmann, K.E. (1993). Biobehavioral organization in securely and insecurely attached infants. Child Developm, 64: 1439–1450.

95. Spitz, R.A.(1965). The First Year of Life: A Psychoanalytic Study of Normal and Deviant Development of Object Relations. New York:International Universities Press, Inc.

96. Spitz, R. A. (1945). Hospitalism: An inquiry into the genesis of psychiatric conditions in early childhood. Psychoanal Study Child, 1: 53–74.

97. Guedeney, A. (1998). Dépression et retrait relationnel chez le jeune enfant: analyse critique de la littérature et propositions. Psychiatrie de l' Enfant, 47: 299–332.

98. Rutter, M., and the English and Romanian Adoptees (ERA) Study Team (1998). Developmental catch-up, and deficit, following adoption after severe global early deprivation. J Child Psychol Psychiatry, 39 (4): 465–476.

99. Kreppner, J.M., O'Connor, T.G., Rutter, M., and the English and Romanian Adoptees (ERA) Study Team (2001). Can inattention/overactivity be an institutional deprivation syndrome? J Abnorm Child Psychol, 29(6): 513–528.

100. Tronick, E., Weinberg, M.K. (1997). Depressed mothers and infants: Failure to form dyadic states of consciousness. In Postpartum Depression and Child Development. New York, Guilford Press. 54–81

101. Tronick, E., Als, H., and Adamson, L. (1978). Structure of early face-to-face communicative interactions. In M. Bullowa (Ed.), Before Speech: The Beginning of Interpersonal Communication (Chpt 17: 349–372). Cambridge, England; Cambridge University Press.

102. Tronick, E., Als, H., and Brazelton, T.B. (1980) The infant's communicative competencies and the achievement of intersubjectivity. In M.R. Key (Ed.), The Relationship of Verbal and Nonverbal Communication (pp. 261–274). The Hague: Mouton.

103. Tronick, E., and Cohn, J.F. (1989). Infant-mother face-to-face interactions: Age and gender differences in coordination and the occurrence of miscoordination. Child Developm, 60: 85–92.

104. Trevarthen, C. (1989). Development of early social interactions and the affective regulation of brain growth. In C. von Euler, H. Lagercrantz, and H. Forssberg (Eds.). The Neurobiology of Early Infant Behavior (pp 191–216). New York, MacMillan.

105. Trevarthen, C. (1990). Growth and education of the hemispheres. In C. Trevarthen (Ed.). Brain Circuits and Functions of the Mind (pp. 334–363). Cambridge, England: Cambridge University Press.

106. Morales,M., Mundy, P., Cowson, M.M., et al. Individual differences in infant attention skills, joint attention, and emotion regulation behaviour. Int J Beh Developm, 29 (3): 259–263.

107. Main, M., and Weston, D.R. (1982). Avoidance of the attachment figure in infancy. In The Place of Attachment in Human Behavior(pp. 31–59). New York: Basics Books.

108. Chance, M.R.A. (1962). An interpretation of some agonistic postures: The role of "cut-off" acts and postures. SympZooSocLondon, 8:71–89.

109. Tinbergen, N., and Moynihan, M. (1952). Head flagging in the black-headed gull: its function and origin. Br Birds, 45: 19–22.

110. Lewis, H.B. (1987). The role of shame in depression over the life span. In H.B. Lewis (Ed.),The Role of Shame in Symptom Formation (Chpt 2: 29–49). Hillsdale, New Jersey:Lawrence Erlbaum, Associates.

111. Kinniburgh, K.J., Blaustein, M., and Spinazzola, J. (2005). Attachment, self-regulation, and competency: A comprehensive framework for children with complex trauma. Psychiatr Ann, 35 (5): 424–430.

112. Cook, A.,Spinnazola, J., Ford, J.,et al (2005). Complex trauma in children and adolescents. Psychiatr Ann, 35 (5), 390–398.

113. Green, J. (2003). Are attachment disorders best seen as social impairment syndromes? Attach Hum Developm, 5 (3): 259–264.

114. Baron-Cohen, S., Leslie, A.M., and Frith, U. (1985). Does the autistic child have a "theory of mind"? Cogn, 21: 37–46.

115. Arranz, E., Artamendi, J., Olabarrieta, F., and Martin, J. (2002). Family context and theory of mind development. Early Child Dev Care, 172 (1): 9–22.

116. Tarullo, A.R., Bruce, J., and Gunnar, M.R. (2007). False belief and emotion understanding in post-institutionalized children. Social Developm, 16: 57–78.

117. Goody, E.N. (1999). Some implications of a social origin of intelligence. In: Goody E.N. (Ed.), Social Intelligence and Interaction: Expressions and Implications of the Social Bias in Human Intelligence. Cambridge, Cambridge University Press. 1–37

118. Hutchins, E., and Hazlehurst, E. (1995). How to invent a shared lexicon: the emergence of shared form-meaning mappings in interaction. In E.N. Goody (Ed.), Social Intelligence and Interaction: Expressions and Implications of the Social Bias in Human Intelligence (Chpt 2: 53–67). Cambridge: Cambridge University Press.

119. Vygotsky, L.S. (1962). Thought and Language. Cambridge: M.I.T. Press.

120. Byrne, R.W., and Whiten, A. (1988). Machiavellian Intelligence: Social Expertise and the Evolution of Intellect in Monkeys, Apes and Humans. Oxford: Clarendon Press.

121. Drew, P. (1999). Interaction sequences and interaction planning. In E.N. Goody (Ed.), Social Intelligence and Interaction: Expressions and Implications of the Social Bias in Human Intelligence (Chpt 5: 111–149). Cambridge: Cambridge University Press.

122. Bjorklund, D. F., and Pelligrini, A. D. (2002). The Origins of Human Nature: Evolutionary Developmental Psychology.Washington, D.C: American Psychological Association.

123. Grossman, K., Grossman, K.E., Spangler, G., Suess, G., and Unzner, L. (1985). Maternal sensitivity and newborn's orientation responses as related to quality of attachment in northern Germany. In I. Bretherton and E. Waters (Eds.), Growing Points of Attachment Theory and Research. Mon Soc for Res Child Developm, 50 (1–2): 233–356.

124. DeVries, M.W. (1984). Temperament and infant mortality among the Masai of East Africa. Am J Psychiatry, 141: 1189–1193.

125. Belsky, J., Steinberg, L., and Draper, P. (1991). Childhood experience, interpersonal development, and reproductive strategy: An evolutionary theory of socialization. Child Developm, 62: 647–670.

126. Trivers, R.L. (1972). Parental Investment and sexual selection. In: Campbell, B. et al (Eds.), Sexual Selection and the Descent of Man: 1871–1971. Chicago, Aldine Publishing Company. 136–179

127. Neel, J.V. (1962). Diabetes Mellitus: A "thrifty" genotype rendered detrimental by "progress"?Am J. Hum Gen, 14: 353–362.

128. Gluckman, P. and Hanson, M. (2005). The Fetal Matrix: Evolution, Development, and Disease. New York: Cambridge University Press.
129. Barker, D.J.P., Forsen, T., Uutela, A., Osmond, C., and Eriksson, J.G. (2001). Size at birth and resilience to effects of poor living conditions in adult life: longitudinal study. Br Med J, 323: 1–5.
130. Barker, D.J.P., Erickson, J.G., Forsen, T. and Osmond, C. (2002). Fetal origins of adult disease: Strength of effects and biological basis. IntJ Epid, 31: 1235–1239.
131. Newman, L. and Mares, S. (2007). Recent advances in the theories of and interventions with attachment disorders. Curr Opin Psychiatry, 20 (4): 343–348.
132. Jernberg, A.M., and Booth, P.B. (2001). Theraplay Second Edition: Helping Parents and Children Build Better Relationships through Attachment-Based Play. San Francisco: Jossey-Bass.
133. Van IJzendoorn, M.H., Juffer, F., and Duyvesteyn, M.G.C. (1995). Breaking the intergenerational cycle of insecure attachment: A review of the effects of attachment-based interventions on maternal sensitivity and infant security. J Child Psychol Psychiatry, 36 (2): 225–248.
134. Marvin, R., Cooper, G., Hoffman, K., and Powell, B. (2002). The Circle of Security Project: Attachment-based intervention with caregiver-pre-school child dyads. Attach Hum Developm, 4 (1): 107–124.
135. Lieberman, A. (2004). Child parent psychotherapy. In: A.J. Sameroff, S.C. McDonough, and K.L. Rosenblum (Eds.), Treating Parent-Infant Relationship Problems: Strategies for Intervention (pp. 97–122). New York: Guilford Press.
136. Hughes, D.A. (2007). Attachment-Focused Family Therapy. New York: W.W. Norton and Company.
137. Purvis, K.B., Cross, D.R., and Sunshine, W.L. (2007). The Connected Child: Bring Hope and Healing to Your Adoptive Family. New York: McGraw Hill.
138. Allen, J.G. (2003). Challenges in treating post-traumatic stress disorder and attachment trauma. Curr Women's Health Rep, 3 (3): 213–220.

About the Author

Daniel Shreeve grew up in a family of writers and in a community of laboratory scientists and their families that filled up and, eventually, transformed the small Long Island village of Bellport. He recalls a carefree and often barefoot childhood during a period when the fields and forests between home and the Great South Bay were open and accessible. His father—a pioneer in nuclear medicine—brought the family to Sweden for a sabbatical, where the author completed high school at Viggbyholmsskolan International School, near Stockholm.

Dr. Shreeve spent his sophomore year abroad at Durham University in England; he graduated Phi Beta Kappa from Washington University in 1971. His doctoral work in ethology included a year of field research at the remote Aleutian island of Adak. As Assistant Professor at Northeast Missouri State University (now Truman University), he taught in his specialty of ethology, but also acquired responsibility for the premedical curriculum in histology and other subjects. This in turn inspired the ambition to study medicine, and subsequently the early interest in ethology found application in the subspecialty of child/adolescent psychiatry.

Dr. Shreeve has served in the US Air Force as Chief of Child/Adolescent Psychiatry at Lackland AFB, and subsequently has provided clinical care in a variety of community and hospital settings. Now that his three sons are grown and independent, he and his wife have moved to Bavaria, Germany, where the he provides child/adolescent psychiatric care to US personnel stationed overseas.

CPSIA information can be obtained at www.ICGtesting.com
Printed in the USA
LVOW070159070412

276588LV00002B/3/P